Also by Terry Reed

The Full Cleveland

THE HIGH SCHOOL REUNION DIET

Younger, Thinner, and Smarter in 30 Days

DAVID COLBERT, MD,
AND TERRY REED

SIMON & SCHUSTER PAPERBACKS
NEW YORK LONDON TORONTO SYDNEY

This publication contains the opinions and ideas of the author. It is sold with the understanding that the author and publisher are not engaged in rendering health services in the book. The reader should consult his or her own medical and health providers as appropriate before adopting any of the suggestions in this book or drawing inferences from it.

The author and publisher specifically disclaim all responsibility for any liability, loss or risk, personal or otherwise, which is incurred as a consequence, directly or indirectly, of the use and application of any of the contents of this book.

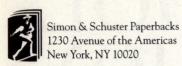

Simon & Schuster Paperbacks
1230 Avenue of the Americas
New York, NY 10020

Copyright © 2010, 2011 by Dr. David Colbert and Terry Reed

All rights reserved, including the right to reproduce this book or portions thereof in any form whatsoever. For information address Simon & Schuster Subsidiary Rights Department, 1230 Avenue of the Americas, New York, NY 10020.

First Simon & Schuster paperback edition March 2011

SIMON & SCHUSTER PAPERBACKS and colophon are registered trademarks of Simon & Schuster, Inc.

For information about special discounts for bulk purchases, please contact Simon & Schuster Special Sales at 1-866-506-1949 or business@simonandschuster.com.

The Simon & Schuster Speakers Bureau can bring authors to your live event. For more information or to book an event contact the Simon & Schuster Speakers Bureau at 1-866-248-3049 or visit our website at www.simonspeakers.com.

Designed by Nancy Singer

Manufactured in the United States of America

1   3   5   7   9   10   8   6   4   2

Library of Congress Cataloging-in-Publication Data
Colbert, David (David A.)
    The high school reunion diet : younger, thinner, and smarter in 30 days / David Colbert and Terry Reed.
        p. cm.
1. Nutrition.   2. Self-care, Health.   I. Reed, Terry, 1958-   II. Title.

RA784.C5665 2011
    613.2'5—dc22   2010046542

ISBN 978-1-4391-2863-3 (pbk)

ISBN 978-1-4391-9979-4 (ebook)

TO MY PARTNER, JP VAN LAERE

MY PARENTS, ED AND DOLLY

MY SIX BROTHERS AND SISTERS

AND THE WONDERFUL
TYSON AND PARIS

Syllabus

Doctor's Note

Health, beauty, beauty, health, youth, beauty . . . I'll tell you a trade secret. It's all the same to us.

"Fusion" has always been our special thing in the dermatology department, where skin health and skin beauty are by nature inseparable. As medical doctors who know how health affects appearance, we are fond of fusion. I think it's even fair to say we've taken our feelings for the word to a whole new level.

I'm the lead physician of a group of New York City doctors who are good at making people look and feel better fast. I'm both a dermatologist and a doctor of internal medicine, and our practice is uncommon in that we mix it up, featuring many specialties that nicely cross-reference one another. We have other dermatologists, other internists, a surgeon, a psychiatrist, an acupuncturist, a fitness expert, and a therapeutic massage therapist. If a new "ist" or an improved technology comes along that can make a major contribution to glowing good health and the consequent great good looks, we'll line up to hear about it. We have skilled medical aestheticians and talented laser technicians to address cosmetic skin care. Keeping us all on track, there's a small cadre of physicians' assistants, many of whom are on leave from NYU

School of Medicine, just down the street at the end of Fifth Avenue. Due to our somewhat unorthodox, multitask-like approach, we've been called a Medical Dream Team in the media, and referred to as Doctor Transformers in O, *The Oprah Magazine*.

But for all that, we didn't set out to design a diet. Frankly, it didn't fit into our modern, advanced-technology theme, or seem to at the time. The inspiration came right behind the realization that patients, even the best and brightest of them, were thinking today's key to "recovering lost youth" was Botox.

glossary of terms: BOTOX

Botox, as most of us know, temporarily smoothes skin and eases wrinkles. Used properly, it's a pretty wonderful drug. You might even call it a Wonder Drug. It's extremely safe, very effective, and if the doctor injecting it has a good eye and a light hand, it definitely has the power to make any face look younger and fresher fast. But that's the extent of its powers.

During the last decade or so (Botox was FDA approved for cosmetic use in 2002), I would sometimes hear from my patients what had prompted them to try Botox. Often, it was because a big event was coming up in their lives and, naturally, they wanted to look their best. Maybe the event was a wedding, a job interview, a red-carpet appearance, or some other significant, and potentially scary, date with destiny. Men and women alike were lining up for the quick cosmetic fix. Yet there was one special occasion that seemed to inspire patients to try Botox so predictably that it made me and my colleagues exchange knowing smiles in the hall. This was shaping up as the mother of all special occasions, sending anyone who could afford it in search of an emergency medical makeover. Another thirty-, or forty-, or fifty-year-old had signed up for the High School Reunion.

———

Apparently, the one thing nobody wants is to flunk the High School Reunion. Nobody wants to be the guy who got fat and old, or the girl who was once such a breath of fresh air, it brought tears to your eyes—or at least does now. Nobody wants to be mistaken for his or her own mother or father from across the gymnasium floor. And of course, what former homecoming queen—or known nerd for that matter—doesn't want the satisfaction of defying all cruel expectation and appearing in front of the old crowd looking as good as, or, unbelievably, *even better* than before? With a reunion looming, the go-to, short-term solution to the long-term problem seemed to be Botox.

Which is asking just a little more of Botox than it can possibly deliver. While Botox does what it does very well, it's not going to make your skin clear and luminous, or your body taut, strong, and shapely, or your eyes bright, or your brain function with youthful speed and clarity. It won't do a thing for your sense of humor, or your hair. The problem with using Botox as a Wonder Drug is that there's a better one out there, and it's even more widely available. You don't need a doctor, it's cost effective, and it doesn't wear off in four to six months. It's food.

I began to ask the cosmetic patients who were looking for reunion-level results the tentative, if leading question: "So what are you eating?"

The inquiry would often draw a blank expression—and it wasn't because of the Botox. (It takes four to nine days for the wrinkle-reducing effect of Botox to kick in—incidentally, about the same amount of time required to detox a patient from a bad diet, reset blood sugar, and initiate a look-good eating plan.)

The answers to this extremely simple but most essential of health and beauty questions—what are you eating?—required a book in rebuttal. But you might be a little surprised at why. On the surface, most of my patients' answers didn't sound all that bad. That is, unless you were a doctor, with the added responsibility of translating them into medical—and cosmetic—consequences.

It wasn't as if our patients were all living on fast food, corn chips, and Cheetos. And it's not that they were so overweight that they truly deserved a sit-down with the doctor. The question of diet had merely come up in relation to the mission: looking good and young fast, including swift repair of the skin. Most of those on this mission were the kind of smart and sophisticated New Yorkers with the money and the motivation to consult a doctor for care for their skin, and many (not all) were making a good-faith effort to eat as well as they knew how.

It's just that by asking The Question, we discovered some gaping holes in our collective nutritional knowledge. Many if not most of those asked were fairly clueless about the physiological effects of sugar, and about where sugar is found, and about what it does to your body and beauty.

Then—even *we* can't blame *everything* on sugar (actually it's sugars, plural, but we'll get to that soon enough)—we also found a general misunderstanding as to the nature and function of carbs and fiber and fat.

And That's Not All

1. We found some serious disconnects in the culture surrounding food, and in what qualifies as convenient, and in what qualifies as cooking.

2. We found that many patients, even though they had heard the word on processed food, weren't always sure when a food (or drink) could be considered processed—and so weren't knowledgeable enough to avoid processed food like their lives depend on it, which we believe they do.

This called for some reeducation.

———

We wrote our diet idea down, and took it upstairs to our CEO to try it out. He had been grumbling that he was overworking, and gaining weight. When he put the pages in his briefcase and then returned from a three-week trip looking fifteen pounds lighter and as many years younger, we felt we were onto something. He, and we, and the patients who followed suit, began to attribute the stunning results less to our skill as MDs and more to their skill as "reeducated" daily dieters.

I won't pretend that all patients were thrilled to hear from their dermatologist that food is the new Wonder Drug. It doesn't sound immediate, and it doesn't sound glamorous. It doesn't even sound verifiable. The only way to prove that diet works cosmetically—even "better than Botox"—is to try it. The patients who did were easily won over. A natural youth and radiance returned to their skin. They lost weight if they needed to, or recontoured their bodies in wondrous ways. They looked younger and happier. Best of all: they felt *great*. And it happened just the way we Americans like it: fast. We named it the High School Reunion Diet, in honor of every one of us. But as we hope you'll see soon enough, you can take the results anywhere.

David Colbert, MD
New York Dermatology Group

Part One

PREP

Orientation

66 In my over twenty years dedicated to providing practical and accessible health information for the masses . . . this simple, sweet, sassy, and sane book delivers the science of looking and feeling good with the easiest, most sensible, how-to advice, tips, and plan that I have come across. Finally, true science and sound advice blend in this book in a way that I can integrate into my life overnight. 99

—Nan-Kirsten Forte, executive vice president, WebMD.com; editor-in-chief, WebMD the Magazine

Let's Get Started

Food is the best medicine we have. It's the key to recovered youth. The radiant skin, the lithe, maybe even ripped body, the good hair, even the confidence, the cool. . . .

If you have thirty days to devote to becoming your own medical dream team, male or female, you can get a lot of that back.

Here's how it works.

The High School Reunion Diet is not a diet book.

It's not a beauty book.

It's not a medical book.

Let's not even worry whether it is a book—or more of a handbook. Our mission is to offer a brief but complete reeducation on the subject of food. When you graduate about thirty days later, you will arrive at the high school reunion looking more like your original young self than you have in years.

———

Contrary to diets past, you're going to accomplish this small medical miracle by eating. Since we last cracked a biology book back in high school, scientists have learned a lot about why we stay hungry, store fat, and gain weight. We've learned with awesome specificity the foods that keep us young and healthy, or make us old and fat. Now we can use those insights to slim down, shape up, get smarter, get cooler, and see our skin become fresh and resilient all over again. And the beauty of it is, all we really have to do is: start eating.

The day when deprivation was the key to weight loss— and when weight loss was the only objective of "dieting"—is so over. Whether you're in it to slim down or just to get back to young, strong, and hot, you'll still need to eat. Quite a bit, in fact. The lessons of *The High School Reunion Diet* are more about what than how much.

We'll be making a big point of encouraging you to eat something we like to call True Food. By this we mean nutrient-rich vegetables, nuts, and fruits, and many other wholesome foods that arrive in their own perfect little natural-born packaging, unadulterated by processing. Food that hasn't been overthought, overhandled, overpackaged, or overengineered. Very likely, it has no label, so doesn't require a lot of tiresome reading. But the real beauty of True Food is, the more of it you eat, the better off you are. Today, it's not discipline that will bring us success in our diet; it's knowledge. And that means, if you want to get back the great body, first you have to feed your head.

Which brings us back to . . . school. If you think you can become your own medical dream team and starve your head, forget it. In fact, let's feed it a little something right now. Recent studies of the health habits of the world's most medically advanced countries reveal that the French in fact eat the most, but Americans are the most obese. Hmmm. Maybe eating the most isn't so bad. Maybe eating less is less relevant than we thought. Maybe it's not how much we eat, but how much of what we eat. Success in diet today is a simple matter of upgrading our Nutritional Intelligence Quotient—here to be known as your NIQ—to match what good medicine now knows about good food.

Based on the results of our many patients who've already benefited, here's roughly what you can expect to achieve with the HSR plan and your new and improved NIQ.

HSRD 101

n this new day of diet, our main job is to bring our heads to the table. In terms of what you'll learn and how you'll utilize the knowledge, here's the way this new kind of diet is designed to go down:

We'll start with a small but bracing appetizer of English (or, "What the Word *Diet* Means"), history ("How We Got Fat and Old"), and science ("True Food: The Good Drug"). Next, in "Too Cool for School," a brief Cheat Sheet will get you started dieting and give you an overview of the process, including general guidelines for Level One (a short detox phase), and Level Two (a maintenance stage).

Next, in the section titled "Drug Test," we'll get to the subject of sugar.

In the "Core" section, we'll quickly upgrade our understanding of carbs, fiber, and fat.

In "International Studies" we'll talk about protein, and in "Home Ec," food culture.

In "The Lists," you'll learn exactly what food to buy and why.

And in "Cafeteria," you'll find a range of suggested recipes that are both simple to make and great to eat. You will be able to tailor the program to suit your individual goals, but basically, our brief but complete reeducation on food is designed to be a group learning experience, and so we're all in this together.

Level One

If you need to lose weight (Level One), you will—and the more you need to lose, the more quickly it will go. You could lose up to eight or ten pounds in the first few weeks—at which point you'll get to rethink some of the Level One restrictions, and maybe some (approved) bread/pasta/rice will be back on your plate. (If you're in it for twenty pounds or more, please first check in with your regular doctor.)

Level Two

Even if you don't need to worry too much or at all about weight loss (Level Two), by eating the recommended foods for thirty days, you will redistribute pounds and trim down at the waist, do mysterious wonders for your skin, and put your visible aging in reverse. You will look younger, and you'll start hearing about it. There's no way this won't happen. And we haven't even mentioned what you've done for your long-term health.

You Be the Dream Team

As you might have suspected, you can't really recapture or keep your good looks without fixing your diet, or look younger without improving your skin and your health, or renew your shape without an inadvertent assist to your overall confidence level. Even if you spend only thirty days eating True Food, you'll still have to tailor your pants so they sit smartly at your waist and not unfashionably at your ankles—which is so grade-school reunion.

———

Back in Iowa where I grew up, my dad was the head coach of a championship high school basketball team—as well as the father of seven—and I feel I put in the hours observing the finer points of the traditional pregame pep talk. So here goes.

Whether you're in this for the good health or the good food or the good looks, whether your goal is to appear at the High School Reunion as the strongest, the smartest, or the most stunning, we know you can pull it off, and we'll be there on the sidelines rooting for you. If you've struggled with weight loss in the past, those days are over. If you've had a strange addiction to foods you know aren't good for your health, that's over too. This time success will be fairly effortless, because you're going to play the game as much with your head as with your heart. A little re-education will go a long way.

Key Lesson

Our bodies are fond of fusion too. Something amiss internally almost always has a way of showing up on the surface. A poor heart begets poor circulation, which begets a poor complexion. Thinning hair can mean an underperforming thyroid. The yellowish fingernails can indicate a lung condition, or a blood-pressure issue. The old style of medicine—treating each issue as distinct, and the cosmetic as distinguished from the medical—is not only too slow, but often, regrettably counterproductive. The HSR system of daily diet is designed to make the entire team work together seamlessly.

Obviously, we believe in the transformative powers of good food, and will do our best to give a convincing medical argument that diet is the most important thing you can do—and the main thing within your own control—to improve your health or beauty or both. But that doesn't mean food can do everything for you all on its own. In a show of good faith, we've listed a few things to help it along . . .

- Check in with your doctor first if you need to lose more than 20 pounds.
- Visit a dermatologist to see if advanced skin care, such as laser treatment, would work for you.
- In the next few weeks try to work less and sleep more.
- Pick up a practical book on daily exercise or head for the gym.
- Make a point of walking places you never thought to walk before.

Let's Review

The key to gaining control of your future internal well-being and your current external beauty is through True Food. So you're going to give it a shot—for 30 days. We're willing to bet you won't stop there. At the very least we promise it'll make you look really, really good for your High School Reunion. It will also educate you, age-proof you, and end up being the most important thing you ever did for your health.

Feed Your Head

66 Well-researched, medically sound, and entirely free of hysteria, *High School Reunion Diet* is much more than a means to an end. It is a lively, smart primer on how to eat, not just for thirty days, but forever. 99

—Siri Hustvedt

If you're a typical American eater, with the habit of consuming first and worrying later, let's assume your head is hungry. So in order to feed the beast, we're going to start with a few small but illuminating lessons in English, History, and Science, which might help our understanding of the awesome medical benefits of True Food.

ENGLISH

Unless you speak ancient Latin, you probably don't instantly recognize that the derivation of the word "diet" translates to mean "daily." This is significant because the whole idea that weight loss

glossary of terms: DIET
The word *diet* doesn't mean "don't."
  The word *diet* doesn't mean "deprivation."
  The word *diet* doesn't mean "hungry."
  Contrary to all we've ever been told about
this short, dreaded, four-letter word, none of the
above is the healthy, the correct, or the sustainable
definition.
  The word *diet*, which comes from the Latin *diet*,
really means "daily." Nothing more formidable,
nothing less familiar.

and improved health would result from interrupting or stopping normal levels of nourishment has been an incorrect assumption of disastrous proportions. In fact, weight control is achieved throught the exact opposite practice of what most of us call "dieting," and is far more likely to happen with the routine consumption of certain foods from a variety of prescribed food groups, like clockwork, every day. This is good news because it means that once we establish the right diet in our daily lives, we'll never have to go on "a diet" again.

The origin of the word *diet* may seem a small point, but medically speaking, it raises an important issue. In the United States, the deprivation long associated with diets billed as weight-loss plans, even many of those designed by medical doctors, has been not only ineffective but often dangerous. Deprivation dieting (including almost every diet you can name, with the most deeply suspect being the no-fat fiasco and the no-carb fiasco) has, in our professional opinion, made *diet* a very bad word.

———

But here, we're just talking daily. As in pleasurable, heartwarming, familiar routine. From now on, the word *diet* will merely refer to the enjoyable four or five times a day we eat, and stay whole, strong, and handsome as a result. Soon it will also mean we deliberately eat some foods and some categories of food often, because this helps to maintain our health and recover our youth.

———

WHAT YOU'LL EAT WHILE YOU DON'T "DIET"

Truth be told, True Food is nothing new. We won't call it old, as that carries unappealing culinary connotations, but does "ancient" work for you? It should, because our early ancestors, the hunter-gatherers, had an admirable body-mass index. They were tall, strong, lean, natural-born Olympians. Long before agriculture was developed (around ten thousand years ago), bringing a more sedentary lifestyle and, soon enough, the refining of foods and the uncivilized use of sugars and other additives, our forefathers ate whole grains, pure fish, grass-fed meat singularly high in protein and low in fat, and fresh, nutrient-packed fruits and vegetables. At the beginning, all food was True Food. On a practical basis, here is how that lifestyle can translate into a diet you can thrive on beautifully today:

Lean meat, preferably organic, is on the menu, including beef, chicken, and turkey (a terrific food that should be

eaten as if every Monday, Wednesday, or Friday were
Thanksgiving Day). We'll also explore the ratios of meat to
plants on your plate, and raise our awareness of complete
protein sources other than meat, because only in America
is the word *meat* synonymous with the word *protein*.

Fish. If you don't like fish, we can talk, but can we interest
you in some shrimp, lobster, scallops, or mussels? One
way or another, you'll be recognizing, and getting, your
essential, youth-boosting omega-3s.

Vegetables. You're going to learn to love your vegetables.
Your body will teach you to. Your brain will wonder what
all the fuss was about in the first place.

Eggs are good, even the yolks. And we'll also unlearn a
few formerly "intuitive" things about what's good and not
good for our hearts.

Nuts are good. So are seeds. If they're not shelled yet, they
also take a while to crack and eat, and as we'll see, slow is
an important factor in weight and youth control.

Water and tea (green, white, and black) are good for the
soul and good for the skin. Coffee is fine, or even better
than fine.

Condiments and spices will rule.

Olive oil will be king, and a benevolent one. You'll find
all foods bow in its presence. On the HSR Diet, it is duly
revered.

Fruit needs an asterisk. The big lesson here is to learn to eat it whole. Fruit without fiber is fructose on speed.

As for **bread and butter**, wait until you hear our feelings on fiber and fat, and are 100 percent sure what the word *whole* means. (It doesn't mean 100 percent.) But no matter what level you are, neither bread nor butter should be a free-for-all.

That's all you need for now to get your head in the game. If you take our advice, you'll be eating quite often (and exceptionally well): three meals a day, plus snacks at least twice to keep you both optimistic and energized. One compelling reason we need to eat enough? Hunger makes us *fat*. You might even say eating *more* is the best way to lose weight—but we don't want to strain our brains just yet.

———

So far, does this sound like a draconian diet? Does this even sound like a *diet*?

Well, we told you about the word. It's a shape-shifter.

Let's Review

That's what the diet is. Now let's reinforce the information by considering what the HSR Diet isn't:

- It isn't high or low fat, high or low carb, high or low protein.
- It isn't a math test, requiring you to measure every gram or ounce, count every calorie, or weigh every pound.

- It won't let you gain back weight that you've lost, or worse, get sick as a result of poor Nutritional IQ.

Key Lessons

Keep in mind that this transformation you'll experience is a perfectly natural biological process. If you can quickly accomplish just a minor shift in intellectual orientation and a few small adjustments in daily eating, then this is what starts happening from a physiological point of view:

1. Your cravings for all the stuff that wasn't real food to start with will simply stop.

2. You'll lose weight if it's warranted, and your skin will begin to bounce back.

3. You won't need to go overboard congratulating yourself for this, because your body will have done the work for you.

4. You can also skip the part where you wrestle with temptation; the right food will take care of that.

There's a reason it's called junk food. If you eat it, you become a "junk*ie*." Bad food is a very real physiological dependence. But you can break the cycle. With the first phase of detox, which is just a matter of days, you will stabilize your blood sugar. It was the roller-coaster up and down of sickeningly high, then crashingly low, blood sugar that was causing the weird cravings and consumption in the first place. That kind of eating more closely resembles the definition of *recreational drug* than of *daily diet*.

That's enough introductory English. Now try some introductory . . .

HISTORY
How We Got Fat and Old

If you're the quick study we think you are, you already realize that all we're recommending is that you recognize and eat real food—and some real foods in particular.

Of course, when we put it *that* way, we seem to be implying that you've been eating fake food, and what's *that* all about?

Listen to history if you want to hasten the youth-recovery process.

In fact, much of the food we've been living on as a nation for several decades (and getting bigger, sadder, and sicker for it) isn't even close to nutritious like food—because it's only "like" food.

But don't sound the alarm because the government already knows. The USDA's stamp of approval, the original Food Guide Pyramid of 1992 that cluelessly promoted processed carbs, helped get us into the health mess we're in. If not exactly upside down, the pyramid was, in effect, on its ear. It called out pasta, cereal, and overrefined grains as particularly commendable, failing to make too much of the fact that those foods are often stripped of their natural nutrients, and doused with sugars during processing. Long story short, sure enough, since then, we've seen an epidemic increase in type 2 diabetes among both adults and children. And, we've gotten eye-poppingly chubbier, too. Fat and sick: these are just two of the effects of eating food that's not really food.

How to Tell True from Fake

The faux food offered in American supermarkets is a credible piece of forgery—or maybe we wouldn't have fallen for it in the first place. It tastes like food, to a reasonable degree, and the package and the TV keep telling us how good for us it is. But even if, as we're sitting enjoying our "enriched!, fortified!, heart-healthy!" breakfast cereal one morning, we decide to take a stab at decoding the contents listed on the back of the box, it's not the word *fake!* that jumps off the page. Actually, our box sounds sort of *smart*. If it *weren't* smart, why would we be so confused?

The label has the heady health jargon of the American food industry on it, the implicit blessing of the U.S. government behind it, even an endearing red heart icon from the venerable American Heart Association (AHA) on it. And in the face of all that heavy credibility, it's tough to keep in mind the fact that this unpronounceable package deal has a good shot at killing us. A trusty rule of thumb? Don't put anything in your mouth if its list of ingredients doesn't roll right off your tongue.

When Food Fell Behind

What else is new? We all agree that spinach is good for us. Popeye made that clear about fifty years ago. Next?

But the thing is, now it's becoming apparent that food isn't the *same* as it was fifty years ago. It's changed quite a lot. And even the good food has changed for the worse. While all that other great medical science was advancing, our nutrition, largely unbeknownst to us, was regressing. The overprocessed, mass-produced, nutrient-depleted, sugar-spiked offerings that now dominate supermarket shelves have almost totally replaced the much healthier diet of our pasts—probably that of our parents and grandparents, and decidedly that of our ancient ancestors—to the point that today, in the United States, our lack of real nutrition has resulted in a very problematic medical situation.

The "Situation"

U.S. diabetes rates have doubled, heart disease is on the rise, cancer rates are at an all-time high. If things proceed the way they're going with type 2 diabetes among ten-year-olds, scientists predict that American parents will soon be outliving their own children. Studies show that 67 percent of all Americans are overweight or obese, and that one out of four children in the United States is overweight or obese. We're being cautious with these numbers; many studies say it's one out of three children. (Be a good scholar and research the epidemic levels of obesity and diabetes on your own—and you'll be as alarmed as we are at the way our food is affecting our health.)

There's a simple medical explanation for the fix we're in. Our food isn't doing what food's supposed to do.

Even our fruits, vegetables, and meats are measurably less nutritious than they were half a century ago. During roughly a fifty-year period (1950–1999), as we produced it in larger quantities, our food experienced a correlative decline in nutritional value. Why? What do the experts say? They say there are several environmental factors, mostly concerning the way we grow, raise, and produce food.

———

It is a difficult and complex business to isolate and quantify exactly which influences are most responsible for the steady decline in our food's nutritional value, but a steady decline it is, as measured by the U.S. Department of Agriculture, which, over a century ago, began tracking such things as how many of our calories come from carbs and sugars, and how many nutrients are delivered in specific foods we raise on American soil. Recent reports continue to indicate that pretty much across the board, good food just isn't quite as good as it used to be. Broccoli, a brilliant food, is not *as* brilliant; it's lost some of its calcium. Chicken has gained fat and calories. Iron content has declined in meat, along with a general loss of the best protein, the good vitamins, and great minerals. In a measurable way, every USDA report shows, there's a little less value there than there was before.

In his enlightening book *In Defense of Food*, Michael Pollan refers to this decline as "the nutritional equivalent of inflation," meaning that to get the same nutritional bang for the buck from a particular food, we have to consume a lot more of it. And this is the latest assessment of the type of food that's still decidedly *good* for us. Once you add food processing to the mix, don't even bother to call it food.

American Malnutrition

If good food can't perform for us as well as it used to, then imagine the consequences of eating fake food. A steady diet of it over decades has left a major portion of our population not just fatter, but also looking older and getting sicker. Somewhat shamefully, despite the excellent Western medicine we keep developing to deal with the ill effects of the fake food, we're doing a worse job of preventing serious disease than almost any other developed nation on the planet.

There's a word for this: *malnutrition*. And counterintuitive as it sounds, you can overeat and still suffer from malnutrition. The empty calories in processed foods keep us fat, and yes, alive, but they don't deliver the nutrients that keep us nourished and healthy (and young). And this seems to be the particular conundrum of the Western diet: plenty to eat, but not enough true food. All the diligent progress in our advanced Western medicine— great drugs, great doctors, great technology—is being steadily undermined by the destructive forces of fake food.

Let's Review

The healthfulness of American food has been in decline. We're all at risk if we don't deal with the realities of our national diet, and we've all suffered to one degree or another from having the wool pulled over our eyes. Even MDs fall victim to deceptive food industry marketing, to the point that many of them are just as confused as anybody about what qualifies as good food or bad food or why. (Vitamin-enriched "fruit beverage," Doc? It's loaded with sugar, so Just Say No.)

Key Lesson

No matter what the all-out health message on the package is telling you, so far, no food science engineer has been able to first take the natural nutrients out of a whole food and then add an approximation of them back in. That's not the way true nutrition, or biology, works.

SCIENCE

True Food: The Good Drug

For health and beauty, simple daily food can act with the healing power of great medicine. Here's just one little example you might take to heart: eating almonds, according to cardiologists, is as effective at lowering bad cholesterol as taking statins. Another: eating cooked tomatoes in one form or another (good news, guys: ketchup counts) several times a week has been shown in studies to slow or reverse the progress of severe prostate cancer in about 45 percent of participating patients. You want more? You'll see plenty of this in "The Lists": foods that have a direct and immediate impact on compromised health, acting every bit as effectively as drugs, and without the side effects. But bad food? It's like a bad drug, carrying dead-serious side effects.

This isn't a discussion about whether or not we still get dessert. We'll all have our dessert again. But what we won't be able to do anymore is ignore where our food is coming from—because there's good evidence that high-yield, "scientifically enhanced," commercial food production from sources such as nutrient-poor

You're So Vain

Can't really believe that what you eat has a direct effect on your so-called youth-recovery? You will by the time you get through The Lists. For now, let's learn a lesson from a quick game of opposites. What if you're one of those people who hasn't a care in the world except your incredible good looks? And what if you turned up your nose at all sound medical advice to use nutrition in the service of those looks? Want to know what you'd look like? It's not a good look for reunion day. Here are some of the more visible symptoms of vitamin and mineral deficiencies in human beings. Imagine entering the old school gymnasium with this set of beauty issues:

- Vitamin A deficiency: acne, dry hair, itching eyes, dry skin, sinus noises, and maybe the flu
- Vitamin B complex deficiency: bad breath, darkened tongue, dry hair, rough skin, tender leg muscles, irritability, memory loss, and confusion
- Vitamin C deficiency: bloody gums, bruises, cavities, muscle loss, and nosebleeds
- Vitamin D deficiency: digestive issues, nervousness, pale skin, and acute sensitivity to pain
- Vitamin E deficiency: hair loss, muscular weakness, and cataracts
- Vitamin K deficiency: brittle bones and bruises

- Folic acid deficiency: sore tongue, depression, anxiety, and fatigue
- Calcium deficiency: brittle fingernails, eczema, tooth decay, and a strange numbness in your arms and legs
- Chromium deficiency: general lack of energy and no school spirit
- Copper deficiency: bone fractures, discolored skin, and oozing sores
- Iron deficiency: brittle nails, dry hair, pale skin, and dizziness
- Magnesium deficiency: broken nails, nervousness, twitching, and sensitivity to noise
- Phosphorus deficiency: tired body, irregular breathing, and rotting teeth
- Potassium deficiency: edema, bad skin, and bad hair
- Sodium deficiency: lethargy, confusion, and vomiting
- Zinc deficiency: brittle nails, poor circulation, splitting hair

Got the picture? Most processed foods have been stripped of the very substances that keep us looking presentable. And "fortified" processed foods lack the crucial delivery system that whole foods provide naturally. That's why we avoid processed—and always eat the opposite.

soils, corn-fed cattle, and big industrial processors, is a huge part of our fat and health problem.

True, if you want to youth-recover and keep it that way, you'll never again get to chow down on low-fat food or fat-free food or food that's been overengineered or tarted up with sugars like HFCS (high-fructose corn syrup). But let's be honest: those things were never much of a party in your mouth to start with, and definitely won't be once you make a daily habit of True Food. That said, you will again be able to eat a chocolate bar or a dish of ice cream or a slab of creamy cheese or a hunk of freshly baked French bread. If, down the line, you gain back a few pounds, you'll have the NIQ to quickly self-correct, on your own tried and true, reliable daily-eating basis, without having to slog through some dreary new diet.

Good food is the medicine. So that makes eating it, as prescribed, the cure.

Part Two

TOO COOL FOR SCHOOL

The High School Reunion Diet Cheat Sheet

> **"** Dr. Colbert's *High School Reunion Diet* is the successful model's secret to glowing skin and a lean, healthy body—which anyone can achieve through proper skin care and his spot-on nutritional advice. I wouldn't walk the runway without it! **"**
>
> —Adriana Lima, Victoria's Secret Angel,
> Maybelline spokesmodel

Everything you need to know to quickly youth-recover can't be learned in diet class. Soon we'll study the physiological effects of food. But first, let's start eating right. Following are the very few school rules.

The HSR Diet is by nature flexible. In our experience, hard-and-fast rules about diet can be more limiting than useful. We hope to steer clear of regimented thinking and instead give you enough information to make the choices that work for you.

As a doctor, I can assure you that you will get back the good body if you take a moment to feed your head. Your head will gradually inform your body that this is the way it's going to be from now on. You'll begin to operate with a little more intellect and a lot more inspiration where food is concerned. That's not to say the process will be slow. I can vouch for this: getting the educational upgrade is not just the best route to success, it's also the fastest.

But that said, we did promise you a "diet," and you're only human, and it's hard to disconnect the old idea of diet from the old idea of being told how and what to eat. So if it will make everyone feel better, let's establish a plan.

Level One is for those who want weight loss and youth recovery combined. At this level, you'll stick to True Food in the most basic preparations, and to lower glycemic foods (see pages 67–70) until you've lost the first five to ten pounds, most likely over the first ten days to two weeks. That will be your detox phase. After that, you can join those already on Level Two foods, which are every bit as good for you, just not as effective for quick weight loss.

Level Two is less restrictive, and geared toward those whose main interests are good health, good body, and great skin. At this level, you'll still stabilize weight and trim down, mostly at your waist. Here you'll have more fruits, more whole grains, including certain approved rice and pasta, and wine with dinner if you want.

————

Okay, now for the quick start. The following simple adjustments in daily diet will automatically set you up for weight loss, reversal of skin aging, better health . . . and a perfectly timed physical transformation that made it all look easy.

Cheat Sheet

1. So long, **"foodstuff."** If we really want to reverse the aging process fast, some things will have to make their departure fast. This will likely include many of the packaged and bottled foods in your house, notably anything with added sugars (fattening for the figure and no friend to the complexion); trans fats (terrible for the heart; and really bad for the skin); bleached-out albino white stuff like white rice, white pasta, and white bread (because the unnatural whiteness is a good indication that the great nutrients have been engineered out).

2. Level One, forget **bread, potatoes,** and all **corn** products for now.

3. Everybody, stop drinking all **colas** and **soft drinks,** including diet sodas, all fruit juices, energy drinks, vitamin drinks, sports drinks, all beer, and hard alcohol. If you need to lose ten pounds or more, hold off on wine until you make the transition to Level Two.

4. Drink a lot of **water**—a lot more than you think you need. You've heard about this, but you're still a little leery of diving

in. You may have also heard that it's a myth and doesn't matter. As a dermatologist and an internist, I would dismiss that. We'll elaborate later, but reach for a glass of pure water right now. Try to avoid plastic bottles if your area has good tap water; many plastic bottles leach chemicals, and of course live forever as landfill waste. Drink six to eight or even more tall glasses of water, depending on your weight and height, starting today, then every day. And sparkling is acceptable; but again, mind the amount of plastic.

5. Use some of your water to wash down a daily **multivitamin** (we're not going to rely on supplements to get our nutrients, but one or two a day makes sense), a **vitamin E 400** (it'll very likely help your skin), and a **vitamin C ester** (we'll get to why we like this one later—but why wait for why?). Take a good-quality **omega-3 fish oil capsule**. Generally you want the omega-3s you get through food and supplements to amount to 1 gram (or 1000 mg) a day. If you have any medical condition at all, first check with your doctor here; we'll discuss how omega-3s can actively treat many illnesses, but should be avoided with a few others.

6. When you go to the store, **go green**. Literally green, as well as good-to-the-environment green. The richer and darker the green, the better the food is for your skin and health. Get used to the color green; it will be the predominant hue on your plate.

7. You can **eat** an apple today, but don't **drink** it. (Best to apply the same rule to your kids, too.)

8. **Berries** (blueberries, raspberries, blackberries, and strawberries). Berries youth-recover us fast, so make a habit of them for thirty days.

9. **Yogurt** eaten every day antiages, but only if you have the pure and natural kind, meaning you start with plain and add sweetness, nuts, or some fruit yourself. Look for Greek yogurt, which is strained longer and therefore thicker. Avoid any yogurt with added sugars. You can sweeten it yourself with a half teaspoon of agave, a natural sweetener with a low Glycemic Index (which we'll discuss next with sugars), or a teaspoon of organic honey. Fresh berries are both sweet and great for your skin. Cinnamon antiages, so maybe try that on a daily basis to flavor your yogurt, too.

10. Unless you're completely averse to the taste of **fish**, increase servings (particularly salmon, mackerel, tuna, and halibut) to at least one meal every other day. The omega-3 fatty acids in fish oil fight inflammation, a condition that can lead to obesity, skin aging, and other conditions. If you can't hack it, take your fish oil capsule. In fact, take it either way.

11. **Olive oil**, which we need in our diets, is an A+ fat. Cook meat and fish in it, and drizzle it on vegetables, starting with your very next meal. Until we discuss Pass-Fail Fats, don't cook or dress foods with anything but.

12. **Spice** it up. Garlic is a natural antioxidant with Top Chef taste, and we encourage liberal use of it. Fresh and dried herbs and spices of all varieties add taste while they simultaneously antiage us, because they're full of the antioxidants that can repair or prevent the kind of damage that causes skin aging and serious medical problems, including diabetes. Pick a few favorite spices and use them when cooking dinner tonight.

13. Go **nuts** (almonds, walnuts, the works). Party-mix on. Make a small bag of nuts today's afternoon snack. For one, the fat slows down feelings of hunger, and will sustain you until dinner. And nuts and seeds feature vitamin E, an antioxidant that aids quick skin repair. Walnuts are another good source of omega-3s.

14. What's for dessert? Nothing yet. But if you want a treat in the meantime, read our fitness expert Kacy Duke's succinct take on sweets, "This Is Your Brain at the Bakery," from her book *The SHOW IT LOVE Workout*.

That's half of the Cheat Sheet. While we take a break and let it sink in, we'll talk a little process. It will help illustrate our indispensable operating principle: Diet Means Daily.

————

Educators—and advertisers—are well aware that we don't get a message until we've heard it more often than we usually wish we had. No matter how smart we are—or how loud or urgent the message—our logical brains learn through repetition. Advertisers call it "frequency," and put big dollars into repeating them-selves. The more often they run their ad, the better chance that you'll be buying their product—perhaps less because you planned on it and more because it has now become oddly irresistible.

Our internal organs work on much the same principle. Keep feeding them a consistent message, and the food to go with it, over and over, and one day soon they'll "get" it, and change will occur. You won't need to make an "effort" to eat a certain way, your body will adapt with ease, in good time. That's one rea-son we've set aside thirty days for your youth-recovery; the body needs a chance to get with the program and catch up with the brain. If you start sending it the right signals now, you'll both be done by reunion day.

The Cheat Sheet Continued

Now here are a few behavioral shifts that should begin happen-ing on a daily basis:

1. **Breakfast, lunch, and dinner.** Hunger makes us fat, so there's no skipping meals in this school. You will even eat a few snacks in between meals, around that time of day when your blood sugar dips and your energy flags. To preview the science for this: blood sugar needs to remain steady for your body's cells to repair themselves and for your metabolism to get on track. That means hunger doesn't help, on any level. And as you've heard, breakfast really is the most important meal; a proper one helps control hun-ger all day. Counterintuitive, of course. But kid you not, eating first thing in the morning is the best way to lose weight.

2. **A new day of shopping.** A regular trip to the farmer's market (or the fresh-food aisle) will do more than anything else to renew the vibrancy of your skin. You'll see why when we itemize the specific health and beauty benefits of the world's best foods. The supermarket is still perfectly acceptable, as long as you navigate it properly. The inner aisles, mostly processed foods, are to be avoided. But the outer aisles, where the fresh vegetables, meat, and dairy are sold, still show plenty of promise. Either way, we prefer locally grown and organic. Remember, high-yield foods grown somewhere faraway—even the vegetables—are measurably less nutritious now than before.

3. **Heavy betting on vegetables.** What do your lovely grandmother and a crusty old sailor man who lives in a garbage can have in common? They both got "Eat Your Spinach" right. Why was that so wise beyond their years? Calorie for calorie, spinach is packed with more nutrients than any other plant—and plants are the glamour food of the new eating plan. Vegetables from the approved list will now take up most of the real estate on your 9-inch plate, whereas meat portions, for most Americans, must be cut down to size—about four to six ounces, max. And any overprocessed food no longer makes an appearance at all.

4. **The classics.** Once you establish a diet of great foods that satisfy your hunger and taste, there's no need for new and different all the time. Even It-Boy and It-Girl chefs are usually cooking the basics. In fact, as you may have guessed, we'd like

you to get slightly repetitive about certain keepers; wild salmon, just for an example, could be eaten four or more times a week. Its omega-3s are great for everything from mood to memory to smooth skin. Canned salmon or tuna is okay, too. Olive oil is a fat, but again, it's an A+ fat, and we'll see why A+ fats should be eaten, not avoided, every day.

5. *Spice* is the spice of life. It's variation in food preparation, not the food item itself, that keeps daily diet lively and interesting. The recommended spices and condiments are rich in the antioxidants that spike taste, improve skin, and age-proof us from the inside out. Perceptible color, aroma, and flavor tip you off that a food is rich in these highly important antioxidants. You'll stock up on basics such as garlic, ginger, basil, oregano, rosemary, and turmeric, and learn to make liberal use of all herbs and spices. They can only improve your looks, your health, and your dish.

The ABC's of Antioxidants

Free radical doesn't refer to the Age of Aquarius-style hippie you aspired to be back in high school. Today's free rad is an unstable molecule that's lost an electron and now intends to glom onto yours. This will cause oxidative damage, mess up your molecules, and maybe alter your cells' DNA. You don't want to hear all the bad things a free rad can do before breakfast, but one of them is major aging, and this you should wake up and fight. Your weapons include a whole arsenal of natural *anti*oxidants that are plentiful in what we call Smart Carbs. You've heard antioxidants touted in skin creams, but the best way to get these fierce warriors into your body is through what you eat. Here are a few of the powerful antioxidants that can make quick work of renewing your cells, repairing your skin, and recovering your looks.

- Allium—in garlic, onions, and scallions
- Anthocyanin—in blueberries, raspberries, strawberries, blackberries, pomegranate, cherries, açaí berries, blood oranges, black beans, and soybeans
- Beta-carotene—in carrots, sweet potatoes, pumpkins, and squash
- Catechins—in green and black tea, dark chocolate, and red wine

- Lutein—in spinach, kale, broccoli, and Brussels sprouts
- Lycopene—in tomatoes, watermelon, and pink grapefruit
- Quercetin—in broccoli, cranberries, onions, and apples
- Resveratrol—in wine

Of course you might already know that the vitamins A, C, and E and the mineral selenium are potent antioxidants, too. Get A from brightly colored fruits and vegetables; C from citrus fruits, tomatoes, peppers, and leafy greens; E from nuts, seeds, whole grains, and greens. Selenium, no slouch, is found in fish, red meat, chicken, and eggs . . . which begs the question, Which comes first from antioxidants, the beauty or the health?

Part Three

DRUG
TEST

The Sugar Addiction Cycle

66 Youth doesn't come in a bottle of Botox but rather in a healthy, nutritional lifestyle. *The High School Reunion Diet* will have you craving fresh foods and shedding pounds just in time for your reunion or any special event where you want to be the best version of yourself. 99

—Jillian Demling,
entertainment editor, *Vogue*

The addictive substance formerly known as sugar is no longer just the pretty white stuff that looks good in our spoon and lights up in our mouth. That's our old, innocent understanding of sugar, left over from the days of cookies and milk at school. The new meaning is complex because it includes the fallout from fifty years of adding various sugars to processed foods.

First, I'll appeal to your vanity. Sugars (that's plural) greatly accelerate skin aging. Sugar triggers a process called glycosyl-

HSRD 101

Take it on faith from a dermatologist: besides sun, *sugars are the main environmental influences that make us look old.*

ation, which causes collagen to cross-link, with the result that the skin becomes stiff, inflexible, and discolored. Have you ever seen the hard, cracked brown crust that burned sugar leaves in the bottom of a pan? That's what eating it does for your skin.

DID YOU KNOW?

Most of us already know that the words *diet* and *sugar* don't go hand in hand. We know that sugar adds calories, pure and simple. But we tend to think of sugar as the mere teaspoon of table sugar (sucrose) we put in our coffee, or are well aware we're getting it in desserts. And that's hardly the case anymore. Now sugars in their various forms are lurking in almost every package on every shelf of your supermarket.

These sugars might be called something else for one reason or another—maybe so you won't think it's, like, sugar—but they're still caloric sweeteners weighing in at about 125 added calories per ounce, and no matter what it's called, your body can't comprehend the label, either, and reads it just like it reads sugar.

That said, we live on sugar. But there's a world of difference between ingesting refined sugars and the glocose that runs our bodies.

glossary of terms:
GLUCOSE/ GLYCOGEN/ GLUCAGON

Food turns to *glucose* inside the body, and glucose is sugar, and we've got to have glucose. It's the source of our energy. It runs our brains and muscles. *Glycogen* is also a form of sugar that we store when we don't burn up the glucose right away. It gets converted back to glucose when we need it. *Glucagons*, another g-word, stimulate the release of glucose when we're hungry and our blood sugar's too low.

If you effectively mainline refined and other added sugars by eating processed foods, you get too much sugar and too quickly, and if you keep doing it over and over, then you're vulnerable to serious threats to your health, and your skin. Too much glucose at a shot causes the pancreas to secrete too much insulin, whose job it is to get the glucose out of the blood and into the brain and muscles. Muscle cells also start to resist storage, and with no-where to go, the glucose gets stored as fat. And if there's too much of *that*, well, now you're at risk for not only unappealing weight gain, but real problems like diabetes and heart disease.

Refined sugars and high-fructose corn syrup and their countless cousins are the killers, and they are dangerous and addictive. Here comes the lesson of the day—in fact, of your life—so study it until you know it cold. It might sound repetitive, but ignore all that. Remember, repetition works.

Key Lesson

The Sugar Addiction Cycle: Most carbohydrates are converted to sugar (glucose) by our bodies, and thus sugar is the source of our energy, and that's all good. But added sugars make for a loaded cocktail. Ingesting sugars as straight sugars (and not in whole foods that will slowly convert to sugar) immediately spikes blood sugar (the happy sugar high). The pancreas oversecretes insulin so the sugar will leave our blood and make our brain and muscles function, which the sugar dutifully does, but in this case, in a dangerous surge. Then, to counteract the wave, the blood sugar dives precipitously, and this creates a strong, biological craving for more sugar (a junkie in search of a fix). To cure the sudden hunger and lack of energy, we desperately seek more of the same: sugar. Eating a lot of sugar hasn't satisfied anything; it's only made us need a lot of sugar. When you habitually eat processed foods with high or even moderate sugar content, you can't easily get off the treadmill. Like any addiction, it becomes a chronic, repetitive cycle.

That would be one thing, if it were harmless. But added sugars play a major role in causing big problems, such as diabetes, heart disease, cancer, obesity, and premature aging. Even so, it's a drug that's not regulated; and special interests chronically lobby against warning consumers about the dangers—while they push for adding even more sugars.

Sugar Sugar

We now have sugar in its many forms in almost all the bottled and packaged foods we consume—including health, vitamin, energy, and fruit drinks, and, believe it or not, even baby formula. Some sugar-laced soft drinks are legally marketed as "health sodas," simply because the marketers cleverly added some vitamins or some trendy antioxidants. Some candies now have added vitamins, which mislead you into thinking you're doing yourself a good turn, or at least a better one. You're not. The added sugars cancel out any nutritional benefits from the added vitamins—not to mention that vitamins are truly bioavailable when enabled by synergists in a whole food. Bottom line, the only way to detox, lose weight, prevent disease, renew your skin, recover your youth, and prolong your life: give every package and bottle the Drug Test (see page 49). Turn it over. See the grams. Stay clean.

If you avoid all processed foods, you can still enjoy a crème brûlée or a chocolate bar on occasion. You've taken sugar out of the drug culture and put it back where it belongs: in dessert after a good meal.

Field Trip!

> **66** Finally, a plan for those who want to look gorgeous quickly and easily while not expecting you to eat nothing but tofu and wheatgrass. **99**

—Mandy Stadtmiller, entertainment writer,
New York Post

This "trip" will take you only as far as the supermarket, but it's still designed to blow your mind. We're going to go out and witness firsthand the wild, widespread, unconscionable use of the addictive and destructive drugs that operate under the many aliases of sugars.

Before we learn its multiple names, understand that some form of added sugar is found in almost all processed foods, which is a key reason they're banned on the HSR Diet and replaced with True Food. These sugars are added during processing for more reasons than the obvious one of jacking up the taste. Besides sweetening (or oversweetening) commercial food, sugars are added to restore lost food structure, texture, and consistency;

to prevent spoiling and ensure longer-than-natural shelf life; for yeast growth in baking; and to control crystallization. Heavy use of sugars for various reasons is an entrenched part of industrial food processing.

DID YOU KNOW?

Refined sugar's none too talented understudy, HFCS (high-fructose corn syrup), is even worse for health, looks, and weight than other sugars. It plays havoc with the very hormones that are supposed to kick in to curb appetite when you've had enough. So if you eat it, or drink it, you don't even know instinctively, as you normally would, when to stop. Yet HFCS is still shame-lessly loaded into snack foods, into drinks and breads and cereals, and even into items enthusiastically advertised with words like "health" and "vitamin" and "smart."

Here's the way to take a stand against all that. No matter what the package says on the front, don't buy it until you check the sugar(s) content on the back. If you must—on rare occasion—eat packaged foods and bottled drinks, look for fewer than 10 or 12 grams of "sugars" per serving. But first get a sense of how much that is.

Also be aware that, in addition to the Nutritional Facts ("the label"), each product lists all the ingredients in the item, and you want to see sugar and its surrogates listed toward the bottom on this ingredients list, definitely not toward the top, because the higher it is on the list, the more predominant the ingredient is. And watch for how many times sugar is listed not only as sugar, but right alongside its multiple aliases, as itemized below. Many

glossary of terms: GRAM

What *is* a gram?

You'll see at the supermarket that the packaged-food labels list sugar content in terms of grams. (And of course, as Americans, grams are our second language, not first.) To get a sense of the plain old American ratios in the packaged food, think of a gram of sugar as about ¼ teaspoon of the table sugar you would put in your cup of coffee. So, to do the math, 50 grams is *12 teaspoons* of sugar in your cup of coffee. You don't put 12 teaspoons of sugar in your cup of coffee—if, for no other reason, because then you'd have to eat it with a fork. Yet you will find this very amount of sugar listed on the back of your average "health" tea drink.

processed foods contain sugar *and* HFCS *and* less familiar caloric sweeteners all in one product—and that adds up to a *ton* of sugar. And while we're on the subject, the more ingredients of any kind listed on the label, the more processed the product doubtlessly is, and that's bad for more reasons than just the added sugars. Stick to foods with as few ingredients as possible, and ideally, those that don't require a label at all. They do exist. Everywhere. An orange or an apple or a bunch of fresh spinach requires no label, because what you see is exactly what you get.

Now let's head to the store and put some of this information to the test.

Drug Test

This isn't a test you'll be taking. It's one you'll be giving. On your field trip to the supermarket, study the backs of the boxes and tubs and cartons and bottles. If you think sugar is listed on the labels simply as "sugar," think again. Here are just some of the many ways the presence of sugars is indicated on the package, in some instances deceiving us, in some just confusing us:

Corn syrup: made from corn and composed mainly of glucose

Dextrose: also derived from corn

Fructose: a sugar in fruits, honey, and root vegetables

Galactose: a sugar in milk products

Glucose: a simple sugar that often bonds with other sugars (Don't let this throw you, but glucose also refers to the sugar produced from foods when they're digested or metabolized. As such, glucose is the body's main energy source. We need glucose, but we need it slow and steady, which is the way it works with whole foods.)

High-fructose corn syrup: a mix of glucose and fructose made from corn; known as HFCS, aka The Devil

Lactose: another sugar found in milk, composed of glucose linked to galactose

Maltose: found in molasses and used in fermentation (beer)

Sucrose: table sugar, bonding fructose and glucose

Is it sweet enough yet?

Apparently the packager doesn't think so. Those are only the dead-giveaway sugars that sport the telling suffix *ose*. Also be aware that processed products are routinely laced with not-so-terrible-sounding . . .

- beet sugar
- brown sugar
- buttered syrup
- cane-juice crystals
- cane sugar
- caramel
- corn syrup solids
- date sugar
- demerara sugar
- dextran
- diatase
- diastatic malt
- ethyl maltol
- free-flowing brown sugars
- fruit juice
- fruit juice concentrate
- glucose solids
- golden sugar
- golden syrup
- grape sugar
- invert sugar
- malt
- maltodextrin
- mannitol
- maple syrup
- molasses
- muscovado or Barbados sugar
- panocha
- powdered or confectioners' sugar
- refiner's syrup
- sorbitol
- sorghum syrup
- treacle
- turbinado sugar
- yellow sugar

So that's a good start. Study the labels carefully, and soon you'll be as alert to stealth sugars as a drug-sniffing dog. And frankly—no offense—that's not a bad comparison. Whether or not you yet fully understand *why* you are being trained to sniff out sugar like it's a deadly substance . . . just go ahead and do the drill, because knowing where sugars are and avoiding them accordingly is the *single most important thing* you can do to protect your health and improve your looks. And part of that, but only part of that, is about losing or avoiding excess weight.

Drug Test Two

That "sugar is the pretty white stuff they put in dessert" way of thinking is beginning to sound a bit naive—in light of what we now know. Right? Let's make sure that's definitely the case. It's your turn to take the Drug Test.

Your New Sugar NIQ

Right now, without thinking too long, name five foods with high sugar content—other than the usual suspects. If you can't remember five from the supermarket, just head to your kitchen; unfortunately, you might be able to complete the assignment in there. Name five *unusual* suspects, products that truly took you by surprise—or at least never before were on your sugar radar screen. For extra credit, list them in descending order, highest to lowest in terms of sugar/danger content.

5.

4.

3.

2.

1.

If you recalled even three foods from the Field Trip that had an alarmingly high sugar content, then your comprehension and memory are already improving your sugar NIQ—and chances for youth-recovery. (Remember, sugars make us look old.) Were any of the following common food items on your list?

Sugars Packaged as Health

1. Did bottled **iced tea** (with a healthy, natural-sounding name, no less) make it onto your list? We assume soda did . . . but, seriously, *tea*? Everybody's telling us to drink tea for the catechins, the flavonoids, the powerful antioxidants said to reduce risk of heart disease and cancers *and* mightily improve our skin.

Yes, but that means pure tea, as in brewed by us, not as in bottled by that mysterious somebody else—who miraculously manages to turn pure tea to pure sugar.

As far as health benefits are concerned, bottled tea is a contradition in terms. Why? It typically has about 50 grams of added sugars, and often one of them is HFCS. That not only cancels the health benefits, it completely reverses them.

———

Check the label. Find a sugar-free tea (not a "diet" one sweetened with aspartame or other artificial sweetener—that's another problem). Good luck; I tried this experiment at the health-conscious deli across Fifth Avenue. Out of about fifty enticing ice tea drinks on display, I found only one that was sugar-free and nondiet. It took me a half hour of label reading. I bought this delightful tea, added a packet of raw sugar, and it was really good. But when I went back for more, it was no longer there. It had been canceled due to lack of interest. You'll probably come to the same conclusion I did: easier to make your own.

2. Did a healthy-looking **yogurt** seem like an unusual suspect? Even as innocuous a flavor as lemon (no crazy "empty calories" in a lemon!) can clock in at around 30 grams of sugars. Why? Because someone *added sugar* to your healthy yogurt and your heavenly lemon and rendered it the opposite of healthy and heavenly even if on its way to your house it got blessed by the pope. Yogurt is a typical stealth place where we find unholy amounts of sugar. Don't stop eating yogurt; just stop buying the kind that has added sugars. If you need sweetness, add agave, honey, real maple syrup, or a little pure raw sugar; and/or throw in some naturally sweet (and impressively beauty-boosting) berries yourself. Greek yogurt, the last time I checked, was still relatively additive-free. Check it yourself when you go to the store.

3. Did a beautiful, "pure," prepared **tomato sauce** speak to you from the shelf? If it did, it should have told you to go home and make your own tomato sauce, because all too often the prepared kind sports about 15-plus totally unnecessary grams of sugars per serving. If you don't have time to make your own, search out one with a low sugar content.

4. Your favorite "natural" **lemonade** weighs in at about 35 grams of sugars and/or contains HFCS. Pomegranate juice? A whopping 50. Same goes for fruit punch, fruit drinks, fruit waters, juice cocktails, juice beverages, juice sprays et al.

5. Your **nutritional bar** came with about 20 grams of sugars, and thus was completely unable to deliver on the *"nutritional."* Same with most sports and energy bars. Always reconcile the front and the back of the package to see if they're on the same page.

6. Your "energy" or "vitamin" or "spa" or "health" water cost you about 32 grams—and, a few minutes later, a definite dip in energy (and a cloying thirst, too). Ditto with most of the sports and smart waters. Try to stick to water that has no marketing adjective on it at all, except maybe spring. Filtered tap water is good.

Bottled water is not regulated, and may contain bacteria, chemicals—even arsenic; city water is quality-controlled. See Recommended Reading for a brilliant book on the subject: *Bottlemania*, by Elizabeth Royte.

7. Your so-called strong-heart **cereal** has about 17 or many more grams of sugars per serving. (What doesn't kill you makes you stronger?)

8. And the instant **oatmeal** you weren't even tempted to eat but did because it was supposed to be good for you had 16 grams of superfluous sugars.

Need we go on? Is *everything* loaded with sugar? Nah, that's just the food and drink that are audacious enough to claim that they'll make us as healthy as a horse.

You may have noticed that we haven't mentioned particular brands while exposing these everyday drug peddlers. That we haven't outed the actual products, just called them by the food categories they fall under. That's because the variation in added sugars from brand to brand isn't often terribly significant. This problem of added sugars has infested almost the entire packaged and prepared food and bottling industries. Sugar is invariably present in processed foods, but you can tell to what degree it's there by doing the Drug Test. The products with very moderate added sugars are definitely worth seeking out. Find a tomato sauce with a conscience, a condiment you enjoy for reasons other than the sugar high, a bottled drink treat with only trace added sugars and absolutely no HFCS.

Key Lesson

Never let someone you can't see decide how sweet it should be.

Known Drug Pushers

Some you will recognize "from the street," some maybe less so. They're all guilty as charged.

- Soda
- Energy and sports drinks
- Bottled iced and "health" teas
- Bottled coffee drinks
- Cappuccinos, lattes, chai, anything with flavored syrup— now featured everywhere from coffee empires to fast-food franchises
- Fruit juices and "100% juice" faux juices and punches and beverages
- Cocktail mixers, including tonic water

(Notice: we haven't even started to *eat* yet.)

- Canned fruit
- Packaged and dried fruit
- Breakfast cereals and instant hot cereals
- Health and sports and energy and nutrition bars
- Packaged diet foods
- Barbecue sauces
- Prepared condiments with added sugars (including ketchup; buy organic)
- Yogurt with flavors or fruit syrups
- Packaged breads, bagels, muffins, rolls, wraps, fruit tarts (especially those with topping or icing)

- Granola and yogurt and soy "health" / candy bars
- Salsa, dips, and chip toppings
- Bottled salad dressings
- Prepared fruit and yogurt smoothies and shakes
- Snack crackers
- Frozen breakfasts, dinners, and pastas
- Instant anythings

Let's Review

Whether weight loss is a necessary part of your plan or not, the added sugars in processed foods must be permanently avoided to protect from serious consequences to long-term health—and visible compromises to the natural beauty of your skin. And that's about all we have to say about sugar.

Recess!

Excellent. You've given your body one of the biggest breaks of its young (and getting younger) life. From this point on, while you're hitting the books, you'll also be adding about ten years to the life of your body, and taking ten away from the way you look.

To fully execute your mental and physical and attitudinal transformation, the next step is to examine some old, entrenched beliefs about carbs, fiber, fat, and a few other things we put in our mouths, which will help turn our thinking around while our bodies get the rest of it right.

Part Four

CORE

Smart Carbs

66 Beauty is my business, and I believe much of my success as a model and actor is due to Dr. Colbert's innovative, noninvasive treatments that give the most natural results possible. 99

—Dara Tomanovich, Face of Olay
Regenerist, Clairol, Max Factor, and Avon

Poor carbs: they've taken an incredible beating. Every fad diet seems to dump all over them, and worse, dump all over *all* of them, as if the carbs from a slice of empty-headed white bread were the same as the carbs from a smart, attractive dish of spinach. The diets do this so you won't get confused and think you can eat carbs on a diet.

We have no intention of similarly underrating your intelligence.

A famous American novelist once said it's the sign of a first-rate mind if you can hold two opposing ideas in it at the same time. He must have been talking about carbs. Carbs are not all the same. They don't look the same, taste the same, or act the same in your body. And even though they've been slandered six ways to Sunday, ignore the hysteria, because we definitely want to make a major point of eating certain carbs on a regular, as in daily, basis, to lose weight and look young.

We call these desirable carbs smart, to distinguish them from the ones that are, well, really very dumb. Smart Carbs aren't just smart; they're the Albert Einsteins of all food groups. These special, brainiac foods include most but not all vegetables, some whole fruits, whole grains, and unadulterated dairy products. That is, intact food that has not been processed to the point it's become deficient in vitamins, minerals, and essential, nutrient-

glossary of terms: CARB

One conceptual problem with carbs is, weight-loss diets are often defined as *high carb* or *low carb* without specifying that at the heart of the matter— all that really counts—is the *kind* of carbs you're eating. With the increasing popularity of low-carb diets, the word *carb* somehow started to stand in for *calorie*, the thing dieters have been told they desperately need to avoid.

A healthful and beauty-boosting daily diet won't trash carbs or suggest you attempt the dangerous high-wire act of going carb-free. *How many* misses the point. The point is to switch to eating the *right* kind of carbs, and to eat them a lot, as in daily.

rich fiber (or fat); loaded with sugars; and bombed with hydrogenated oils (trans fat) to compensate for lost consistency or taste. Smart Carbs are key to a youth-recovery diet, and eaten regularly will actively *help*—not just *not hurt*—both weight loss and skin repair.

———

The HSR Diet grades carbs based on their natural ability to energize, nourish, and stabilize blood sugar; to repair and renew skin; to curb cravings and satisfy appetite. Carbohydrates (the word comes from carbon/hydrogen/oxygen—so you should hear the word *plant* in there somewhere) are one of three main nutrients in foods. One of only three. That means they are very, very important. They are converted during digestion to glucose, which we now know is the sugar that runs our bodies and that we can't survive without.

DID YOU KNOW?

Carbs are essential—nonnegotiable—if you want to continue to live. Carbs are found in fruits, vegetables, whole-grain breads, milk products, and sugars. They are of course also found in baked goods, pastries, junk food, bleached pasta, white rice, and processed foods—which is where their reputation went south. But that last list of losers excludes Smart Carbs.

———

One thing you can do to determine if carbs will act smart or not so smart in your system is to consider where they stand on the Glycemic Index.

GI 101

The Glycemic Index is a ranking device developed by scientists that measures foods containing carbs according to how quickly the carbs turn to glucose in our blood. (You probably guessed that the *gly* preface in *Glycemic*, similar to the one in *glucose*, refers to sugar.)

A carb on the Glycemic Index is ranked relative to pure glucose, which is given the rating 100. A carb with a low glycemic rating will cause a less dramatic rise and fall in blood sugar than a carb with a high glycemic rating. Remember, this is good, because steady blood sugar, among other things, is the perfect way to get our bodies functioning efficiently and to regulate our appetites.

Key Lesson

Smart Carbs—the ones that contribute to total health, weight loss, reduced risk of diabetes and heart attack, *and* skin health and beauty—are the ones that rank low on the Glycemic Index (the GI). They win this ranking (it's like golf; low is good) because they naturally produce only small fluctuations in blood sugar and insulin levels. All glucose produces some rise and fall, but it's the relative degree that makes all the difference. Smart Carbs are brilliant foods, and for you to be as smart, and to get yourself all due reflected glory, you can study where they stand on the Glycemic Index and then start thinking and eating accordingly.

———

The Glycemic Index, as you'll see, is a fairly straightforward business, but there is an asterisk. A good glycemic rating doesn't mean that just because there's a decent number next to the food on the index that that's the end of that and you don't have to use your head anymore when choosing carbs. Some of the rankings on the index seem entirely logical. For example, oat bran bread has a 68 GI (medium), and a French baguette has a 136 GI (very high).

That's a big difference, but not a big surprise.

You more or less already knew the score there. Oat bran, good. Baguette, bad. So it makes perfect sense that their glycemic scores diverge.

But sponge cake and cooked carrots have about the *same* GI ratings, 66 and 68; and it's obviously not a mark of genius to dine on sponge cake instead of carrots. There are several other factors, including nutrients and fiber, to be taken into consideration.

Still, since the key to our success here is to achieve steady blood sugar (again, for weight control *and* skin repair), it makes sense to take the Glycemic Index seriously as a reference when choosing carbs, and to trade in your habitual high-GI carbs for lower ones. Doing it now will make a marked difference in thirty days.

Here's the range, and again, the number is relative to pure glucose—or a piece of white bread—at a GI of 100. Remember, it indicates the precipitousness of the rise in blood sugar—and keeping it steady is the name of the game.

Highest GI: 100 plus

High GI: 68 plus

Medium GI: 56–69

Low GI: 55 or less

Great GI: 20 or less

Next is a list of common foods, ranked by their Glycemic Index. You can't memorize them all, and the numbers aren't set in stone, but you will get the idea of how certain groups of foods rate. High-glycemic foods should be avoided for health and beauty reasons on the daily diet permanently, except for a well-earned dessert or the occasional splurge. Low and lowest ones should be eaten often for both weight and beauty control.

Glycemic Index

Bakery Products

Angel food cake	95	Cookies	77–115
Croissant	96	Cupcake	104
Doughnuts	98–108	Muffins	70–146
Pancakes and waffles	96–146	Pop-Tart	100
Pound cake	77	Sponge cake	66

Breads

Bagel	103	Baguette	136
English muffin	110	Hamburger bun	87
Kaiser roll	105	Multigrain	61
Oat bran	68	Pita	82
Poori	117	Rye	71
Rye, light	97	Tortilla, corn	74
Tortilla, wheat	40	Wheat bread	76
White bread	100	White, enriched	110

Cereals and Grains

All-Bran	60	Barley, pearled	36
Barley, rolled	72	Bran flakes	106
Cereal bars	80–110	Cheerios	106
Cornflakes	116	Couscous	93
Cream of Wheat	105	Froot Loops	98
Grape-Nuts	102	Muesli	77
Oat bran	78	Raisin bran	87
Rice, brown	72	Rice, instant	124
Rice, long-grain	80	Rice, white	90–99
Rice Chex	127	Rice Krispies	117
Seminola	78	Shredded Wheat	107
Special K	98	Total	109

Dairy

Ice cream	89–97	Milk, fat free	46
Milk, low-fat chocolate	49	Milk, whole	38
Soy milk	46–63	Yogurt	51
Yogurt, low-fat fruit	47	Yogurt drink, fruit	58

Drinks (nonalcoholic)

Apple juice	57	Coca-Cola	90
Cranberry juice cocktail	97	Gatorade	111
Grapefruit juice	70	Orange juice	81
Quik Chocolate	76		

Fruits

Apple	34	Apricots, dried	44
Apricots, raw	82	Banana	73
Cherries	32	Dates	147
Grapefruit	36	Grapes	66
Kiwi	75	Orange	60
Peach	60	Pear	47
Pineapple	94	Strawberries	57
Watermelon	103		

Legumes

Beans, baked	69	Beans, butter	43
Chickpeas	39	Chickpeas, canned	60
Fava	113	Kidney	42
Kidney, canned	74	Lentils	41
Lima beans	46	Soya	20

Nuts

Cashews	31	Peanuts	21

(Note: almonds and walnuts, two major List foods, have only trace GI)

Pasta			
Fettuccine	57	Gnocchi	97
Linguine	74	Macaroni	67
Mac and cheese	92	Spaghetti	64
Spaghetti, wheat	46		
Vegetables (High GI)			
Carrots	68	Corn, sweet	86
Parsnips	139	Peas	68
Potato, baked	158	Potato, boiled	72
Potato, French fried	107	Potato, instant mashed	123
Potato, mashed	105	Potato, new	81
Pumpkin	107		
Vegetables (Low–medium GI)			
Tomatoes	23	Sweet Potato	63
Yams	53		

Vegetables (Great GI): The Smartest Carbs			
Artichoke	Arugula	Asparagus	Beets
Broccoli	Brussels sprouts	Cabbage	Cauliflower
Celery	Chard	Collard greens	Cucumbers
Escarole	Eggplant	Green beans	Kale
Lettuce	Mushrooms	Mustard greens	Okra
Peppers	Snow peas	Spinach	Summer squash
Turnips	Watercress	Zucchini	

Snacks, Sugars, and Miscellaneous			
Agave	22	Corn chips	103
Fruit bars	71	Honey	83
Hummus	9	Jelly beans	78
Maltose (beer)	150	Mars Bar	93
M&M, peanut	47	Popcorn	89
Potato chips	77	PowerBar	75
Pretzels	119	Rice cracker	130
Snickers bar	97	Solid chocolate bar	70
Soups	63–90	Table sugar	92

Let's Review

If you study the GI and get strategic about it, you may notice that it's pretty easy to substitute low-GI foods for high. It's well worth the switch, because the accumulated payoff in terms of health and looks is substantial. For instance, you won't suffer much if you habitually swap out a baked potato (158 GI) for a sweet potato (63) or a yam (53), but you've made a significantly healthier and skinnier choice. An apple will cost you only 34 GIs (and has all kinds of good things for your skin in its skin), whereas a glass of apple juice starts at 56, and many of the nutrients in the apple and its skin are MIA. Stellar vegetables such as broccoli, spinach, sprouts, lettuce, squash, and many others have a negligible glycemic impact, but if you opt for peas or corn, you're tipping the plus-68 point; and if it's mostly potatoes you so unwisely selected instead of something good and low, you're topping out at well over 100 on the chart—just through the seemingly innocent act of eating a vegetable.

———

That's one way to keep blood sugar at a steady level: mind the food's natural-born GI. But if that was all there was to it, the game would be over. The game's not over, because carbs, even smart ones, can't operate all on their own. They may be super-stars, but they are still just one of the starters on a championship team. Fiber and fat are major players too. . . .

Fiber Forever

> **66** Now I can FINALLY go to a high school reunion! The only problem is—everyone else will have read it, too! **99**
>
> —Richard Thomas, actor, *The Waltons*

Fiber is like the school crossing guard. It doesn't get enough respect, even though it has an extremely important job to do. Little fiber is standing in the middle of the road holding the big sign telling sugar to slow the hell down. Fiber rules. Because its presence is key to determining how fast it all turns to sugar.

To get a sense of the interstate system within our bodies: the process of converting the food into glucose starts in our mouths, with our saliva, and continues with the muscular churning and chemical breakdown via gastric acid once the food arrives in our stomachs. While this "road work" is going on, our bodies are revved up and raring to get at the glucose. But we already know that steady—not lurching, much less pedal-to-the-metal—blood sugar is the secret to the kind of smooth ride that keeps us healthy and young. To maintain steady, we need to both mind the *amount* of sugar *and* check its speed. One simple way to do the latter is to eat food rich in fiber.

DID YOU KNOW?

The very presence of fiber slows the conversion to sugar. It goes like this. We eat the food to get the glucose into our bloodstream, but before the glucose is released, the stomach has to use the anatomical jackhammer and complete the sizable task of methodically breaking the food into its components. If there's fiber present, that's a bigger job. The stomach will have to separate the fiber from the sugar and the starch. This work takes time—lots more time than if the fiber weren't present—and thus the rate of sugar absorption is slowed. (Like single file in a traffic jam, the stomach releases the sugar in steady increments as it "processes" the food.) Because of the presence of fiber, our blood sugar surges less, then stops. The stop is TBA because that's when we feel an overwhelming physiological need to do just about anything to gun the engine and go for broke: get sugar. And our heads won't be thinking "steamed broccoli" when that's the state of road rage our bodies are in.

———

To ensure effortless control over the rate of digestion, one of the simplest things to do is to make a point of ingesting food that is structured in its very nature to take its time. To revisit the *good food is good medicine* metaphor, you might even call it time-release food.

Conversely, what if the fiber's already been mostly removed

from the food? Think of the innocent orange. This is a wonderfully healthy food that can easily be corrupted through processing. The pulp in a whole orange is the fruit's fiber. There's lots of fructose (sugar) in fruit, but the natural fiber will slow down the sugar's assault on our systems. But if you juice the orange before it even gets to your mouth, you've pulverized the pulp (the fiber), taken the work away from the stomach, and subjected your bloodstream to straight sugar—and we know you know by now, that's not good. Check back to the Glycemic Index. The whole orange gets a 60, but the orange juice gets an 80. It's the same food; it just took longer for your body to eat. And slow and steady is the whole plan.

So if you want wholesome OJ on a regular basis, have a fresh, whole orange and let your mouth and stomach do the juicing. And of course that same rule applies to apples, and grapes, and cranberries, and pomegranates, and other fruit, too. To fully appreciate this, read the sugar content on the typical bottle or carton of juice. Even if the product is HFCS-free, and self-described as 100 percent pure (we'll talk about the misleading use of *pure* and other marketing buzzwords), it is still very high in sugar, especially if all the fiber that was in the pulp has been taken somewhere out back behind the Dumpster, never to be seen again.

Key Lesson

As a general rule, the less pureed or pulverized any food is, the better it is for our health and beauty. A daily diet of real, whole True Food, replete with Smart Carbs, brings the fiber back in and so naturally curbs the release of sugar, and thus the cravings for more sugar. This helps control weight *and* slow the aging process, which is why you start looking better almost immediately.

About That Bread . . .

Given some of the misinformation you've been fed over the years, you've probably been operating under the principle that bread and cereal, and other mid-level IQ carbs like pasta and rice, while not exactly slimming, are not unhealthy for us. After all, pasta and rice come from two of the world's healthiest cuisines (we'll examine this further in International Studies). And the French, they're not fat—and aren't they all about bread . . . *under* the butter and cheese?

Before we get to the rest of the world, first let's just take a bite out of American bread. Bread isn't bad. But you can't call our national loaf—white bread—"bread." (Same goes for its evil twin, the famous fast-food bun.)

We don't have to look too closely to see that white bread doesn't really resemble what you'd call good bread. That's because that beige mound that allows you to eat your burger with your hands has been processed to within an inch of its life. This has given it the hefty glycemic rating of 100, the very same as straight glucose.

The food engineers who thought up white bread took the wheat, pounded it into over-refined flour, blasted out all the good nutrients, erased any trace of fiber, and mashed and molded the pale, mealy result into a soft, malleable slice or all-too-aptly-shaped hot dog or hamburger or hoagie holder. Then they added sugar or

HFCS to mask the fact that it no longer had any taste, and piled on the preservatives to ensure that it would enjoy a long, pointless shelf life. They stuffed it in a clear plastic bag and described it with adjectives that seem, upon contemplation, flat-out overconfident, like *wonder*. By the time you eat a blob of white bread, it has no nutritional value whatsoever. As food, it's entirely useless. As poison, it shows potential.

Key Lesson

We mentioned the advent of agriculture, and how, funny thing, that historical turn of events coincided with the advent of humans complaining about being fat. But, long story short, bread, if you're slim enough to eat it, has got to be as close to the original grain as possible. And it has to be free of added sugars and HFCS.

This means the bread feels rough and hearty, and looks brown and healthy. That look and feel and natural hue are an indication that the food still has fiber in it, which gives it not only a distinctive, wholesome touch and taste, but also a big, important job to do once it's entered your mouth.

———

Good color and good texture also distinguish whole-wheat pasta and nonwhite rice. You may have tried these in the past and not liked them, but try again, because the taste has been improved. Or maybe it's just that our palates have been improved. If you ask me, it's hard to taste the difference anymore between bleached pasta and whole-wheat pasta—especially under a great sauce (the vegetable and protein component that are supposed to be the major portion of the dish anyway). But whether it's been overrefined or not has a huge influence on your long-term weight and health. You know why now: the fiber that slows the sugar, and the nutrients that remain snugly intact inside.

DID YOU KNOW?

The presence of good nutrients (the kind that save your health and looks) is often indicated by good *color*. The red in tomatoes is from lycopene. The yellow in squash and mango, from lutein. The orange in sweet potatoes, from carotene.

So if white bread serves any purpose at all, at least it's a succinct visual reminder of why not to eat processed food. You can tell just by looking at it that the nutrients are gone.

After all, what in nature grows flawlessly white, is so spineless it dissolves in your mouth and retreats under your thumb, and arrives on the planet in the form of identical molded slices or domes? Can you picture a field of white breads, blowing gently in the breeze? Can you imagine it hanging off trees in an orchard or swimming in a school of white breads in a sylvan lake?

If you cannot fathom a food's logical origins, or for the life of you figure how it came to be on your plate, there's a good chance it's not nearly up to the job of nourishing you. And because of what's come out of it and gone into it to make it look the way it does, it could cause serious health complications if consumed regularly, over time.

Key Lesson

Don't eat white bread, white rice, white pasta, et al. They do not pass the True Food authenticity test.

Deconstructing "Whole"

Once you know better than to buy white, it's still a case of buyer beware. Unless you're getting your bread at the local bakery, buying it (or anything) in the prefab bag has become an increasingly risky business. Bread makers have jumped on the health-promotion bandwagon, invariably stressing how 100 percent their product is, and invariably neglecting to add that this and other enticing marketing ploys mean exactly nothing in terms of nutrition.

FYI AND YOUR NIQ

A whole grain is a little powerhouse of antioxidants, lignans, phenolic acids, phytoestrogens, and other phytochemicals. The whole grain delivers micronutrients such as folic acid, magnesium, and vitamin E. It's chock-full of fiber. Think weight control, cancer prevention, long-term protection against heart disease and diabetes, and swift yet natural renewal of your skin. With all that hanging in the balance, maybe it's worth decoding the label after all.

contradiction in terms:

WHOLE & 100%

The word *whole* does not mean the same as *100%*. If a product claims it's *100% multigrain*, that sounds pretty good from a nutritional standpoint. But in fact the product could have very little *whole* grain in it at all. Read carefully, because all that *100% multi* really means is that the bread has 100 percent of different grains, which may or may not include a whole lot of whole ones. It's the word *whole* that really matters. *Multi*grains do nothing for us unless they're whole.

Whole, in relation to grain foods, is a word that hasn't become 100 percent meaningless yet—but stand by. For the time being, it's a very important word to look for. You want whole grains for the reasons we've already discussed—because breaking and busting and smashing the grain knocks out the true nutrition. But if the grain is allowed to remain whole, then the food stays dense with nutrients, rich in fiber and vitamins and antioxidants, complex carbs and minerals. Whole wheat is a whole grain. If the package says *100% whole wheat*, and then, flipping it over, you see *whole-wheat flour* listed as the first, meaning predominant, ingredient, you're in business. (That is, provided there's no HFCS—or other added sugars.)

Same with whole oats and rye and pumpernickel. However, if the package slyly claims it's *Made with Whole Grain*, it may as well claim it's *Made with Snake Oil*, because this product *might* contain enough whole grain to make it worth eating, or it *might* contain 1 percent of whole grain and 99 percent of not-whole grain. Either way, it still gets to say it's *made with* whole grain. If it says it's made with *wheat flour* as opposed to *whole-wheat flour*, also deep-six it, because wheat flour is *overrefined flour* (not the same as *whole-wheat flour*), and overrefined flour is not good for us. The world *whole* has to be in front of the word *wheat*.

Key Lesson

No matter how convincing the front of the package is, turn it over and look at the list of ingredients on the back. Just like the situation with sugar, the front and back of the package don't necessarily tell the same story, and it's somehow become *our* job to determine if they are in outright contradiction to each other. If

Humpty Dumpty 101

Other grains that are safely whole enough to keep you healthy include barley, brown rice, buckwheat, millet, quinoa, sorghum, and wild rice. These whole grains deliver the very sort of complex nutritional package that all the king's horses and all the king's men couldn't put together again.

whole is the first word you see on the back of the bread, that's a good sign that the product is in earnest and not just messing with your head.

Cereal

Another peculiarly national "foodstuff" (besides bread-by-the-slice) is American breakfast cereal. Our supermarket aisles are stuffed with cereal boxes, and the countless cardboard containers clamor for our love and attention by making all kinds of wild health declarations, which have come a long, winding way from the day when it was just about whether Mikey Likes It.

We hate to take a hard line against such an American icon as breakfast cereal, and we also love the familiar mascots that have been selling us our morning meal on television for more than fifty years. But we took an oath to do no harm, and our best medical advice is to ignore almost all marketing angles and don't eat it—at least not until it passes the Front and Back tests we now will use on everything that comes in a box, a bag, or a bottle.

DID YOU KNOW?

Precious few of our favorite cereals can deliver the health benefits they so loudly claim. Many of them are so overprocessed, they lack fiber, and then have such ungodly amounts of added sugars that they not only hurt us, they make us hungry. This is definitely not the way to start the day—or any diet. Add the sugar rush of a glass of fruit juice, and you can begin to understand why so many of us, adults and children, are sick with diet-related disease, or just too fat.

Convenience is not a good enough excuse. The simple bowl of cereal becomes a lot less simple and convenient when you understand its complicity in causing epidemic levels of type 2 diabetes in adults and children. Being overweight from overconsumption of stealth sugars—and lack of real fiber at the start of the day, when it's most important for your daily hunger control—leads to innumerable, extremely inconvenient health complications, including the very heart disease the "heart-healthy" cereals displaying the AHA stamp of approval promised to protect you from.

Key Lesson

Study that box of cereal carefully before you buy. If sugars are listed in the contents, especially near the top of the list, put it back on the shelf. If the list is too long, put it back on the shelf. It indicates you're getting much more than you bargained for, and plenty of it is bad for your health. There are some cereals in a box (or a bag) that are relatively additive-free, contain whole grains, and deliver good fiber. But you're going to have to be very alert to hype as you hunt them down.

Take-Home Assignment

This next suggestion about our beloved breakfast in a bowl may not sound quick or convenient or even American, but it's a little change that pays off big in the long run. Feed yourself (and your

First-Term Reality Check

You forgot why you even enrolled in school, or what was supposed to happen while you're here? Relax, it's already happening. Just the few changes you've already made in eating and educating will have a dramatic effect on your beauty and health. Here are some of the subjects your body's been addressing while your brain's been working on backup:

- **Chemistry.** The elimination of added sugars is stabilizing your blood sugar along with impulse control. This detox phase is resulting in weight loss, improved complexion, revived strength, stamina, mental clarity, and flexibility.
- **Geography.** You've located the farmer's market near you because it sells the true thing, fresher and often cheaper, too. You've found it's quite pleasant to walk there, and many other places you go.
- **Art.** You're developing your natural eye for proportion and color, dominated by deep green. Consciously or less so, you're redesigning the look of your meals.
- **Biology.** The nutrients you're receiving from whole, unprocessed foods are stopping or slowing oxidative damage throughout your body, protecting you from serious illnesses like heart disease, diabetes, and cancer, and swiftly repairing the natural clarity and resilience of your skin.

kids) oatmeal—not the quickie kind; rather, the slow-cooking, steel-cut, possibly Irish, whole-oat variety that takes about thirty minutes to prepare. You can start it when you wake up, then eat it when you're out of the shower. Even instant oatmeal doesn't cut it—why? You know already: it's been processed. The processing has already "conveniently" broken down the fiber for you, and brought in the sugar, sending its GI rating through the roof. *Slow* is the goal. *Instant* anything is the fast track to fat and unhealthy.

Pass-Fail Fats

66 The models I work with live a majority of their visible lives in only lingerie. Enlightened choices in diet and nutrition provided by Dr. Colbert's *High School Reunion Diet* help maintain their shape, confidence, and heavenly glow. 99

—Todd Thomas, designer,
Victoria's Secret Fashion Show

Once there was a talented yet misrepresented team player. Despite his natural abilities, he was summarily dismissed from his starting position, unfairly benched for a number of years, cruelly bumped to the minor leagues, and finally banned from playing the game. During his long, dark years of exile, he was relentlessly trash-talked by experts and amateurs alike. But now, against all odds, his fate appears to be changing. Soon, his reputation will be resurrected, and then he can resume his rightful place as starting player, key team member, and reigning superstar.

This is the story of fat. They took the right fat out, and put the wrong fat in.

DID YOU KNOW?

Fat is an essential nutrient, and another vital food component (besides fiber) that slows down the absorption of sugar. This makes it a *desirable* addition to meals and in-between snacks. It's an effective hunger-stopper. So it helps to have fat in your diet, for one because its presence will help keep blood sugar steady, therefore making it longer until you're hungry and sooner until you're healthy. Fat is even famous (in some circles) for its ability to satiate. In fact, there's an old diet trick: have a little fat before dinner (French dieters put a dab of butter under the tongue) and you'll eat less automatically.

But just because fat is an essential nutrient, that is not to say that *all fats* are essential nutrients. Far from it. Fat has a range of behavior that goes from very very good . . . to when she was bad she was horrid.

Key Lesson

There are different types of fat; some are great for you and some are actively dangerous. *This next point is central to your reeducation, and it's an "essential" medical fact:*

It's the *type* of fat that matters.

We've been hearing, ever since we can remember, that fat threatens not only our physiques but also our coronary and cosmetic health. And it well may have simplified things, to have fat always playing the bad guy. And then to have engineered, "low-fat" foods ride in to save the day, promising that we could, in effect, have our cake and eat it, too.

Low- and no-fat-labeled foods suggest we can remove the fat but still get the taste. But often these foods have added sugars or man-made trans fat to compensate for the taste or consistency that left with the True Fat. In any case, the whole low fat craze is cluelessly encouraging us to avoid fat while fat, believe it or not, is a *most essential part* of a healthy daily diet.

It's the type of fat that matters.

Therefore, you have to be able to tell the difference between them. There are fats that will keep us young, slim, and healthy, and there are fats that will make us fat, old, and sick. Some fats should be embraced forever and some fats should be dismissed for good. Healthy fats and lean proteins will *assist* in weight reduction and youth-recovery. They can *improve* blood cholesterol, *lower* blood pressure, *ease* inflammation (the overactivity of the immune system linked to heart disease, stroke, diabetes, and skin aging) and other chronic conditions. It's not a matter of not eating fat; it's a matter of knowing which fats to eat.

But first, know that the worst of the bad fats is truly Public Enemy Number One. It's trans fat. As we'll see, trans fat is not a real fat, it's a fake one. You can use margarine as an example for now. Another fat, which has gotten a bad rap in the past that it doesn't fully deserve, is saturated fat. You can use butter as an example for now. And we'll definitely learn why butter is better for us than margarine, so we won't make that costly mistake again.

A Brief History of Fat

Despite the fact that there was *little evidence ever* to recommend low-fat and no-fat foods and diet as a way of life, through a massive antifat initiative that developed in response to disturbing national health statistics, that's what happened, and the thinking was based on the misguided notion that a low- to no-fat diet helped prevent or treat heart disease.

Now we know it simply isn't so. The prominent Women's Health Initiative trial published in the *Journal of American Medicine* in 2006 revealed that, over a period of eight years, a low-fat diet lowered incidence of cardio, stroke, and heart disease in almost fifty thousand women studied *not at all.*

Seriously. Turns out, health, heart, and otherwise, is not really about the *amount* of fat you eat, but the *kind* of fat you eat. And this goes for weight loss and skin health, too. What's more, the A+ Fats help *prevent* disease, and the Fats That Fail *cause* it. Unfortunately, the fats we switched to in the effort to protect our hearts and lose weight were the Fats That Fail. But we didn't understand that then, because we had already made a really bad call on the one thing we fear more than fat: cholesterol.

Mistaking dietary cholesterol as the cause of heart disease is how we got stranded by the low-fat diet debacle in the first place. So now, if we want to get our bodies right, we have to get this fact into our heads: the main thing that impacts blood cholesterol is

glossary of terms:
CHOLESTEROL

The reason scientists called the situation with fat wrong for so long is, in a word, cholesterol. The word *cholesterol* engenders fear across the board. But upon further examination, we realize that that word, not unlike *carbohydrate*, has been confused—with itself. There are two kinds of cholesterol: dietary and blood. Because they have the same last name (like Smart Carbs and Dumb Carbs do), for years, we've believed that high cholesterol in the diet caused high cholesterol in the blood. But *the fact is, dietary cholesterol doesn't directly relate to blood cholesterol* in healthy people. (To further confuse you and the issue, with certain medical conditions, like diabetes, it *can* relate, so in such cases, diet must be overseen by the attending doctor.)

the *type of fat* in the daily diet, not the amount of cholesterol consumed in food.

True, this new understanding of fat seems to fly in the face of everything we've believed all along: that all dietary fat directly and adversely affects waistline and cholesterol levels. But it gets even better. It's not just the good news that the right fats *don't hurt*. It's also the even better news that they actually *help* healthy cholesterol in the blood get rid of the bad cholesterol. And then the best news follows. The great fats can *reverse* the damage the bad fats have done. Again: they *improve* blood cholesterol, *lower* blood pressure, and *ease* inflammation.

You want to raise your healthy cholesterol levels (HDL: high-density lipoproteins) to assist in the fight against the unhealthy (LDL: low-density lipoproteins). Cooking with the great fats, dressing vegetables and salads and breads with them, having the fish full of them, and eating the nuts rich in them all help to *improve* your health, *not just not hurt it.*

FAT 101

In terms of losing weight, as mentioned, the great fats also perform a key fat function: satiety. Replace the bad fats in your diet with them and you're already well on your way to the perfect win-win of weight control and youth-recovery.

In terms of the crucial ways they affect our health and looks, here then is the final Pass-Fail report card on fats.

Fail: Trans Fats

Mostly man-made, trans fats were the Frankenstein monster of a food industry that discovered more than a hundred years ago that by adding hydrogen gas to unsaturated fats food makers could prevent spoiling, retard breakdown during heating, and turn liquid oil to solid for ease in use, transport, and storage. It gave the food a longer shelf life. Trans fats also saved the food makers money, in that the concocted solid fat was cheaper and lasted longer than the natural solid animal fat.

The food packagers loved it. Trans fats invaded commercial processing, inevitably used in the United States in commercial baked goods, snack foods, margarines, fast foods, in fried foods from French fries to doughnuts, and in almost any packaged food looking for an unnaturally long shelf life, which most of them were.

DID YOU KNOW?

The words *partially hydrogenated vegetable oil* or *vegetable shortening* were the ones that typically indicated the presence of trans fats.

It didn't sound terrible. In fact, it all seemed like a really good idea at the time. Didn't a product made from vegetable oil *sound* healthier than one made from butter and lard from animals? And didn't it make food look perkier longer? Yes, but it was one of the major nutritional mistakes in the entire history of food.

In the early 1980s (closing in on a century after the thinking-up of trans fats), some researchers began suspecting that trans fats were worse on the heart, the blood vessels, and general health than the once-demonized saturated fats they often replaced. One tip-off was, Americans were eating them constantly in packaged and fast foods, and Americans seemed to be getting sicker, particularly with coronary disease and diabetes. And Americans were getting fat. Store-bought, packaged foodstuff like cookies (about 95 percent of them) and crackers (about 100 percent of them) and snack packs and flavored popcorn and chips and prepared breakfast foods, and tons-of-fun-sounding after-school treats (and the list goes on) all contained trans fats. Our supermarkets, like our waistlines, were bursting at the seams with them.

———

By the nineties, twenty some years of unchecked trans fats later, research was supporting the thinking that trans fats had adverse effects on the health and the heart, and had been a serious health threat from the get-go. The research was finding that trans fats raised bad cholesterol and lowered good cholesterol. Trans fats increased the risk of developing heart disease and stroke. They were also associated with increased risk of type 2 diabetes.

This sorry report card made them far worse than the supposedly heart-disease-causing saturated fats they had ridden in to replace. Turns out, *any* fat is better than trans fat. Butter, lard, and tallow used in cooking and serving are safer. Solid vegetable oils like coconut oil and palm oil are safer. Fully hydrogenated (as opposed to partially hydrogenated) vegetable oils render a saturated fat without trans fat and thus are safer.

But the safest choices in cooking and eating are the liquid fruit and vegetable oils like olive, canola, and soy. Since these oils don't take high heat as well, fast-food outlets have been slow to deep-six the trans fats from the deep fryer in favor of them. Some cities (New York was the first) have either banned trans fats in restaurants and school cafeterias and stores selling prepared foods, or else have required menus to list to what degree they're there. Many other cities are following suit. As for the situation at the supermarket, since now the amount of trans fat must be listed on the label, food packagers are fairly willing to replace them with safer fats, because it's just bad PR to put the equivalent of a loaded gun in your product.

Take-Home Assignment

At home, throw away the margarine or other trans fats in a tub (vegetable shortening, butter substitutes, partially hydrogenated vegetable oils) and substitute olive oil and even some butter. (Note: now there are trans fat-free margarines made from a blend of healthful oils, and these are safe and acceptable.) Look for trans fats on the labels; if they're there, put the item back on the shelf. Avoid trans fats in restaurants and fast-food outlets. The only thing worse than you using them yourself is allowing someone else to do it for you—and losing all sense of how much of this unnatural, artery-clogging fat you really consume.

3, Four, 6, Eight . . . Who Do We Appreciate?

There have been many studies done on the beauty of omega-3s. Perhaps you're already well aware. But to review, the benefits of getting regular omega-3s in the proper balance to another essential fatty acid, omega-6, are . . . what's the medical term? Mind-blowing.

Omega-3s have been shown to very happily affect the heart. They reduce plaque, decrease blood clotting, have a positive effect on triglycerides (blood fat), reduce blood pressure, inflammation, and risk of death by heart attack.

Omega-3s have also been shown effective in treating or reducing risk of diabetes; insulin resistance; cancers of the colon, prostate, and breast; arthritis; ulcerative colitis; and osteoporosis. For the skin, they can treat psoriasis and acne. For the overweight, they can help blood sugar control. Even depression can be treated with omega-3s, as they boost serotonin and dopamine levels in the brain. And that's just a taste, because there's lots more.*

Omega-6, that other well-known essential fatty acid, is where the balancing act comes in. If one EFA is too high, it may compromise the effectiveness of the other. Americans typically get too much 6, and too little 3. Omega-6 is found in meat, and we tend to get plenty of that; 6 is also found in the safflower, soybean, and corn oils that are often used in processed food—and we traditionally tend to get plenty of that. You don't want to top off on the 6s at the expense of the 3s.

Omega-3s are found in fatty fish such as mackerel, salmon, tuna, lake trout, sardines, and herring, in flaxseed oil, canola oil, walnuts, and some vegetables.

Are you still taking that fish oil capsule we recommended on the Cheat Sheet? Beautiful. Benefits can usually be seen in two to three weeks.

*Omega-3s have also been shown to have positive results in treating or preventing arthritis, osteoporosis, bipolar disorder, bowel disorders, ADHD, wound healing, asthma, macular degeneration, and stress. If you have any of the above conditions, consult with your doctor about omega-3s.

DID YOU KNOW?

If it's still hard to buy the notion that all fat's not bad for you, consider these stats. Fifty years ago, almost *half* the calories in our diet came from healthy oils and natural fats, and we weighed less—*and* we had a much lower rate of heart disease and diabetes. Over the years, due largely to the freak-out over fat and its supposed complicity in causing weight gain and heart disease, our fat consumption *decreased* by about a third, but our disease rates went up by even more.

So even if it doesn't sound so logical (that's you're *old* nutritional logic rearing its ugly head), use good fats daily and forgo foods that have been marketed as lower in fat or fat-free. They may contain dangerous additives, and besides, "fat-free" is not how we lose weight. Why? You now know the answer: *It's the type of fat that matters.*

Deep Background on Body Fat: Lipoproteins

All foods contain some fat, even carrots, and all bodies have some fat, even the flawlessly toned and athletic. Body fat is present under our skin to make it soft and supple as subcutaneous fat, and in our blood as both lipoproteins and triglycerides (these in more of a storage mode). Fat is an essential source of energy and a key nutrient.

So banish the thought that all fat is undesirable and see how it works and how it can work for you.

Since fat and cholesterol can't dissolve in blood, they get carried around in particles covered with protein called lipoproteins, which are able to enter the blood. (As we know from liposuction, *lipo* stands for fat.) The L after *HD* (high-density) or *LD* (low-density) reported by your doctor after your annual checkup stands for lipoprotein.

The type of lipoproteins you want a lot of are the high-density HDL. The type you want to keep low are the low-density LDL. Here's the difference:

- Low-density lipoproteins (LDL) transport cholesterol *from the liver* to the rest of the body. Cells latch onto these lipoproteins and take fat and cholesterol. When there is too much LDL cholesterol in the blood, these particles can form deposits— you've heard of plaque—in the walls of the coronary and other arteries. The plaque on the arterial wall literally narrows the artery and limits the flow of blood. When plaque breaks apart, it can cause a heart attack or stroke.

- High-density lipoproteins (HDL) take cholesterol *from the bloodstream* and *from artery walls* and carry it back *to the liver* for disposal. HDL protects blood, in essence by transporting it and cleaning it.

  The lower your LDL and the higher your HDL, the better your defenses against heart and other chronic disease. Diets rich in A+ Fats—

polyunsaturated and monounsaturated—automatically decrease levels of LDL, and increase HDL in the blood. Healthy fats should make up about 25 percent of your daily calories.

- *Memorize this.* It's the *type of fat* that matters. It's the *type of fat* that affects the amount of total and LDL cholesterol in the blood. Cholesterol in food *does not directly correlate* with blood cholesterol (again, except with some medical conditions, like diabetes, in which case you ask the doctor). A+ Fats don't hurt, but actively *help* your health and your heart.

Pass: Saturated Fats

You've probably heard some nasty things about saturated fats. But unlike the trans fats, saturated fats need not be banished, just limited to reasonable levels. Saturated fats are found in meats and dairy products, and overconsumption can be controlled by choosing lean cuts of meat, grass-fed beef, changing the proportion of meat-to-veg on your plate, and using a light hand with dairy fat. But keep in mind that the saturated fat in a pat of butter is far healthier than the equivalent amount of trans fats in a spread of margarine or other "butterlike" substance. And again the old diet trick: A pat of butter will make the bread it's spread on ultimately *less* fattening, not more, despite the added calories. A dipping in olive oil would make it even *more* less fattening. Fat satiates, and thus slows our hunger and satisfies our appetites.

A+: Unsaturated Fats

Now for the good part. The great fats are true beauty food, not only because they help your skin but also because they contribute mightily to general glowing good health. If you haven't already, then start immediately to very deliberately make the switch to the category of fats we call A+ Fats. These are the excellent, monounsaturated fats and polyunsaturated fats that deliver both great taste and great heart. These are the fats you should embrace in your daily diet because they will (1) keep you trim and healthy and (2) make you more fun to look at.

If you seriously don't yet know and love the world's most beautiful fat, which should have a revered place on your kitchen shelf (and on your bread or vegetables, in place of the butter, and definitely instead of the butter-pretender), then this could be why you've been struggling to understand your weight. Olive oil has been dubbed a superfood. But you wouldn't be overdoing it if you called it a celestial food, as its effect on your health can be transcendent. The fatty acids in olive oil have been shown to not only control weight but also help brain function, improve arterial function (i.e., declog arteries), reduce blood pressure, fight depression, and improve skin.

That amounts to a high-end health insurance policy you can afford, and would be crazy to live without. Health-protecting fatty acids are also found in oily fish, canola oil, nut oils, oil-rich avocados, and flaxseeds.

As for the polyunsaturated fats, you can find them in sesame oils and vegetable oils (not partially hydrogenated) and they, too, will help control appetite and improve health.

Fat Crib Sheet

We've totally lost the trans fats. Here again, for easy reference, are the intelligent choices.

A+ Fats: unsaturated fats—monounsaturated and polyunsaturated—actively *improve* your health and your looks. These A+ Fats mostly come from plant foods, such as vegetable oils, nuts, and seeds. They are liquid (as opposed to solid like trans fats) at room temperature. Think of mono and poly as a set of twins, quite similar but not the same.

Get your monounsaturated fats in

- Olive oil
- Canola oil
- Peanut oil
- Fish oils
- Nuts
- Avocados
- Seeds (pumpkin and sesame)

Get your polyunsaturated fats from

- Vegetable and sesame oils
- Soybeans
- Sunflower and corn oils
- Flaxseeds

Note: Omega-3 fatty acids are one type of polyunsaturated fat. These EFAs are the ones with so many proven health benefits—especially for the heart, as they've been shown to decrease risk of coronary disease and may lower blood pressure. Again, they are found in fatty fish such as salmon and mackerel as well as in flaxseeds and walnuts.

Most research shows we don't get enough of the great unsaturated fats on a daily basis in our diets. Start routinely putting them in your meals and soon, not only do health risks decrease but age-related decline (particularly arterial aging) begins to reverse. Food starts to taste better, too.

Pass: saturated fats—though they're not as bad as once believed, and butter beats margarine by a mile (in the aforementioned nurses' study, those who ate margarine as opposed to butter were at a much *higher* risk of heart disease and stroke), it still makes sense to choose unsaturated fats over saturated on a routine basis. Since our bodies make it, we don't really require saturated fat in our diet, and too much can present a threat to cardiovascular health. Red meat and dairy fats are therefore to be watched—and the era when the steak is as big as your head is over forever.

The recommended meat portion on your plate now should be about 4 to 6 ounces, or a piece about the size of the palm of your hand. That's less than we used to eat, and you want to opt for omega-3-rich fish at least three times a week. But still, you can enjoy saturated fats if you can learn to make sense of them and moderate, and scale portions down from out-of-this-world, supersized.

Saturated fats are found in

- Meat
- Seafood
- Whole-dairy products and reduced-fat dairy
- Some plant oils, like coconut and palm

International Studies

"Are you *really* ready to see all those people again? A new outfit and a spray tan aren't going to cut it! Read this book and get yourself together so that you aren't caught sobbing at your locker again."

—Mike Albo, writer and performer

This will be quick. It's about Le Burger, us, and the rest of the world.

———

Remember Samuel L. Jackson and John Travolta's priceless exchange in *Pulp Fiction* about the Royale with cheese? It was hilarious at the time to imagine a fast-food franchise selling Le Big Mac in the heart of Paris. It's not so funny now, when you consider that there's a McDonald's du Louvre, or that trans fats (born in the USA) are being increasingly used worldwide, especially in developing countries, where cheaper, partially hydro-

101

genated oils are replacing far healthier, traditional oils. These global shifts in daily diet are linked to new, epidemic levels of cardiovascular disease. Even cancer rates in other countries are associated with the slow but steady adoption of the weirdly addictive "Western" diet.

Our export of Le Burger isn't the only way we bungled our end of the foreign exchange. Even the way we *imported* foods has often ended up doing us more harm than good. There's nothing wrong with the foods we adopted—at least not in the healthful context of their originating cuisines. But we *changed* the context: we supersized (made it bigger) and Americanized (made it faster). Since we only learn from our mistakes, here are three you'll recognize:

- **Italian pasta**. In Italy, it's one small course of many in a diverse diet that includes fish, meat, and A+ Fats like olive oil. Here, we liked it so much, it became the whole meal.
- **Asian rice**. In most of Asia, it's served in a small rice bowl, with lots of vegetables, bite-size pieces of meat or healthy-fat fish, or other star proteins like soy. Here, it's served on a 12-inch dinner plate under U.S.-size portions of everything else.
- **Mexican tortilla**. In Mexico, it's a healthy, low-GI staple (especially the wheat variety, with a rating of only 40), served with a complete protein—the combo of rice and beans. Here, it's a trans fat-fried chip dipped in processed salsa, or a "nacho" smothered in faux cheese: either way, an international disaster.

Yes, we're a big, young, exuberant country. But we do have a tendency to pile on. This is where we're going to grow up, get humble, and learn to allow other, older, wiser cuisines to inform and improve our own.

Which brings us back to that American icon: Le Burger.

One big cultural difference between us and almost everyone else on the planet is the way we use meat in our daily diet. And we use meat the way we do because somewhere in our heart of hearts we truly believe that meat is the only really legitimate source of protein. And that is really just not right.

How the World Rocks Protein

You might well argue that protein is out of place in International Studies. Protein is a major food group, on the estimable, life-sustaining level of carbs and fat—and it belongs in the *real* curriculum, right?

Frankly: not anymore.

Don't get us wrong; protein in your daily diet is just as important as it ever was. Next to water, protein is the most predominant substance in the body, and it must be replenished daily, because about half of what we need to sustain ourselves and stay alive comes through food. But let's face it, this is America, and lack of protein is not really our problem.

In the USA, where persuasive food industry marketing has managed to make the word *protein* mean exactly the same as the word *meat*, we don't lack protein. And the way we use this protein source (meat) is a key difference between our increasingly dangerous diet and that of the rest of the world.

Key Lesson

Just as *carb* is not synonymous with *cake*, and *fat* is not synonymous with *fattening, protein* is not synonymous with *meat*. Though meat is an excellent source of complete protein, all protein doesn't come from meat or other animal products, and there are other very good sources. Some vegetables (spinach springs to mind) have so much protein they can put Le Burger to shame. We'll hear about these star-quality foods soon in The Lists. In the meantime, and to explain why protein landed like extra credit in the international section, other developed countries have something we desperately need: a sense of proportion about meat. In fact, *the main thing we want to ease away from in order to stay young and healthy is a diet overdominated by animal products.*

Taking a Cue from International Cuisine

The best food in the world proves that you can still have a wildly successful cuisine and a delicious diet if you cut the meat portion down to size. In some cultures (notably, Asian), meat or fish is considered more like the garnish—the way we Americans look at a prize tomato, or an appealing-enough pickle, on our plate. Vegetables and sauce and grains are the real stars of the Asian meal; the meat is just an intriguing side.

Granted, we're Americans, and we're never going to think of our steak in quite the same way we think of our tomato. Actually, we want 'em both, and we want 'em both big. But if you start to at least entertain the idea that protein also comes from plants, and that the best fats come from plants, you can begin to shift your perspective to that of the far healthier global one—where meat just isn't allowed to overwhelm the rest of the diet. (Remember your vanity: we're talking places where the people stay slim, look good into old age, and live longer than we do.) In all the world's best cooking, a little meat can go a long way. So seriously consider the way they do it in:

Italian cuisine. One of the world's most popular cuisines, the Italian meals are a masterpiece of structure: first the appetizer (antipasto), often including a protein like cheese; then the primo piatto, which is pasta or rice; the secondo piatto, which is meat or fish; then the dolce, which will probably include fruit. A staple here is the A+ fat in olive oil. And though courses keep coming, the portions are small—and all perfectly healthful and satisfying.

French cuisine. Cheese, wine, butter, cream . . . slim, stylish, intelligent, urbane. Apparently fat isn't *that* bad for you, as long as you take it in context (and it's true fat and not faux fat). In France, vegetables, fish, meat, and fruit are all served, but the French have a national knack for perfect proportion. Even though they are brilliant at pastries, the French don't eat them in the outré portions we do. They buy them at the bakery, not the supermarket, and they use real butter and good oils instead of trans fats in cooking and baking. A pat of butter or a square of chocolate are de rigueur, but the food is fresh, the cooking is ex-quisite, and the meal is long.

Chinese cuisine. The world's largest cuisine—feeding a third of the people on the planet. No slab of meat is served here; in the Chinese tradition, every diner is served a bowl of rice, and the other dishes—meat, vegetables, and fish—are served on main dishes that are shared by the table. The meat pieces are small so they can be retrieved adroitly from the communal dishes with chopsticks.

Indian cuisine. Spicy hot, inventive, and loved worldwide, this hugely diverse cuisine is based in vegetables, legumes, and sauce, with animal products—lamb, beef, chicken, and fish—treated mostly as an accent.

Thai cuisine. A masterful use of spices in sauces makes this one of the world's most popular; like other Asian-based cuisines, it features rice and vegetables, with fish, seafood, and some beef—used but not overused.

Japanese cuisine. An extremely healthy cuisine that's based in seasonality, it provides rich protein and nutrients through fish, vegetables, rice, and soy products such as fermented soy, miso, and soy sauce—delivering excellent, nonanimal protein that's low in calories, high in calcium and iron, and proven to lower bad cholesterol.

Spanish cuisine. Beautifully light, down-to-earth, and healthful, olive oil and garlic are basics for cooking vegetables, fish, seafood, and meat. Wine and fruit are part of the daily menu, as is a long, by our standards, lunch. It's probably not irrelevant to weight and health here that the main meal is traditionally in the middle of the day, and the lighter one's at night.

Mexican cuisine. Influenced by both the Spanish and French, it's high in taste, artful in spice, and sufficient in protein without overdoing the meat component, which usually comes cut up, and thus sized down. Rice and beans combined, like meat, is a complete protein (the kind we need for sustenance on a daily basis), and the combo is a low-cost but nutritious national staple.

Greek cuisine. The Mediterranean diet has been extolled for its curative effect on heart health (shown in recent studies to clearly reverse cardiovascular disease), but that aside, it tastes great, with a little bit of Turkey and Italy at play. Olive oil cooks and dresses a variety of vegetables, and then there's the rich source of fish and seafood from the Mediterranean Sea.

Lebanese cuisine. Very big on vegetables, using minimal meat, this exotic Mediterranean-influenced Middle Eastern cuisine is full of rich taste. Beans and lentils are featured and are a great source of protein. It also stars fresh fish and shellfish from the sea, and fresh fruit from the favorable climate of the region.

———

Now keep the big world in mind as we walk down the hall to Home Ec. . . .

Home Ec

At the beginning, we promised you some fusion. And we've just read how worldwide, we all pretty much eat the same foods; we just eat them in a somewhat different way. If you eliminate trans fat and processed food from the equation (as you personally already have), in any culture of notable cuisine, including ours, there's meat, poultry, fish, dairy, grains, nuts, fruits, and vegetables to combine into a daily diet.

But that said, there's more to food than food. There's the culture around food—including the way in which we grow and raise it, the way we package it, the way we shop for it, and the manner in which we prepare it. Since we've gone this far toward an intellectual upgrade, maybe it wouldn't hurt to examine just three latent nutritional disconnects that still stand in the way of our complete American-as-apple-pie health and youth makeover.

"Fast" Food

At one point in time the very notion would have been incomprehensible to an Italian, or a Greek, or a French man or woman—and, by the way, would have sent your great-great-grandmother straight to the fainting couch. *Lunch* elsewhere in the world can still easily take two hours. Meals are meant as a delectable pleasure, not just a dire necessity, and are savored, at length, among family and friends, rather than shoveled in solo and best forgotten.

DID YOU KNOW?

The *slow* approach to food has socio-psychological benefits, but also physiological ones (like the *slow* approach to glucose). The result of eating *longer* is not only greater pleasure; it actually, medically, means eating *less*.

———

Your body is designed to let you know you're not hungry anymore once you've eaten enough. When you approach satiety, your brain starts sending otu chemicals that amout to a 20-Minute Warning. When these chemicals start to kick in, you'll begin to get the message, Okay, thanks for lunch, you can stop eating now. The only problem with this perfect plan is: 20 minutes!? Are you kidding? In America, lunch is over by then. We tend to pound down food so fast, our brains literally don't have time to deliver the Stop Eating signal.

We would do well to eat meals like the rest of the world—with passion and appreciation is invariably better. And it's always a good sign when you have someone else around with whom to share the experience.

Eating together, at least one meal, preferably dinner, is so important on so many levels, I should call in the staff psychiatrist to write a sidebar about it. In the meantime, just from a pure physical-health perspective, we eat better when we eat together. For one, someone has put his or her time and thought into preparing a balanced meal—which doesn't usually fall together just so when dining at the door to the refrigerator. And we eat more slowly when we eat with family or friends—if only because you can't talk with your mouth full. This doesn't mean if you're eating alone you can't eat like a king. It's the ritual of shopping, preparing, and enjoying—polished off with a little bit of gratitude—that has actual *physiological* benefits. This nurturing process just isn't part of the fast-food experience, whether it's at the franchise or not.

Speed Shopping

In France and Italy and other world-beating food cultures, grocery shopping is like American baseball: a sacred national pastime. Here, we tend to shop for food like it's the great supermarket giveaway: grab as much as you can as fast as you can and race with the cart to the cashier. No wonder: the supermarket, with its boxes and boxes and tubs and cartons, can be a soul-sucking experience. One cure for this is to shop somewhere other than, or in addition to, the supermarket, i.e., the fresh-food or farmer's market.

The farmer's market turns food shopping into a whole new ball game. Once you locate it, you might even find yourself walking there—and that's good for the body, good for the spirit, and not bad for the environment. You might find yourself talking there, connecting with other people—shoppers and sellers, growers and cooks—trading comments on the fresh, locally grown food that's for sale, and sharing in an important communal experience. You might find you're more selective there, that you linger and look because the food is so attractive there. You might get inspired to take this beautiful food home and do right by it by cooking it with a little more love than you could muster for the assembly-line stuff at the supermarket. And please don't say . . .

"I Can't Cook"

Assuming you're not a danger to yourself and others around an open flame, you *can* cook. Can you pour a few tablespoons of olive oil into a skillet and gently heat it up? Can you peel a few garlic cloves and mince them and toss them in? Can you add the spinach you bought at the farmer's market and rinsed under the faucet to the skillet with the garlic, sprinkle in some salt and grind in pepper, and shake and stir a few minutes until the spinach wilts? Not only can you cook, you can cook *Italian*.

This is all that healthful cooking has to be: about three steps, out of the bag, under the water, into the pan. Everything good and basic can be approached with this kind of simplicity and clarity. And basic food, cooked simply, will improve your health and your looks faster and surer than anything else. Friends of mine, an Italian couple who can cook like rock stars and often host big dinners for friends, assure me that if we rookies spend more than thirty minutes making a meal, we're not only wasting our time, we're "torturing" our food. So as long as we're more than willing to eat Italian, we may as well dip into some of their context, too: characterized by grace and ease and camaraderie.

Take-Home Assignment

There are many great cookbooks that feature the basic art of Italian, French, Mediterranean, Asian, and other world-class cooking. Sure, you can overachieve just like an American and create a lemon angel food soufflé cake or a fish en croûte à la Julia Child. But save that kind of artistry for special occasions. On a daily basis, in our American kitchens, as we'll soon discover, there's no reason any of us can't cook simple, luscious food that will indulge our palates as it sustains health, as it promotes wholesome good looks and a happy, healthy, long life. For centuries, in cultures much older than ours, it's been the way of the world.

Now for what you're going to bring home, and how you're going to put it in the pan: "The Lists" and "The Meals."

Part Five

CAFETERIA

The Lists

The following lists aren't suggesting you limit your diet to only the items named. But these are the True Foods to make friends with, for life. Generally, to recover youth and keep it that way, you want to consume and combine, and incorporate into your permanent daily lifestyle. So for easy reference and fast youth-recovery, here are . . . the lists.

Vegetables

Beans and legumes

Fruit

Fish, meat, and poultry

Nuts and seeds

Dairy

Grains

Spices and herbs

Honey and chocolate (optional)

Tea, coffee (optional)

Wine (optional)

Water (not optional)

It doesn't sound like much. Of course, like the six or so numbers on a Lotto ticket, there are millions of variables therein. But forget the million for now; you can do that on your own time, after the required thirty days. Within each category, there are many foods that are such clear winners and that so "miraculously" upgrade your system, they should be eaten a lot . . . a lot lot . . . as in every day, when indicated. And though by no means are these the only excellent choices within each category, we've called out some of the best ones for improving your weight, health, and beauty in the blink of an eye.

Vegetables

This is the top list. Vegetables are plants. That sounds remarkably obvious. Less so is the increasingly compelling fact that plants are the healthiest things on the planet to eat, both for us and for the environment. It stands to reason that the major shift we want to make is toward a diet dominated by plants. Vegetables, legumes, whole grains, and fruits are all plants. We'll get to the other plants soon, but calorie for calorie, the most nutrient-packed foods—and the quickest way to lose weight and years—are the star vegetables, and now you'll know exactly why:

Broccoli. For its anticancer capabilities, particularly against gastric and prostate. For its vitamins A, C, K, B_6, E, its potassium, calcium, folate, and fiber. At 45 calories a cup, you cannot get fat on it. Good for blood cholesterol, blood pressure, and bones. Cauliflower is no lightweight, either. Switch them around, but eat one or the other every day or every other day for now. Even if you hate it, eat it. Dash on some soy sauce (low sodium, with no added sugar or HFCS) and learn to love about the best preventive medicine on planet earth.

Brussels sprouts. For the C, K, A, protein, and omega-3s, just to scratch the surface. Iron, protein, and calcium, too. Plus these sprouts have the good glucosinates—think immune system and antioxidant defense. Anticancer capabilities include breast and colorectal. Eat them if you tend to use high heat in cooking meat; somehow (studies show) they help you counteract the possible carcinogens.

Cabbage. 'Cause it's got the C we need from food every day. It's also got the Bs and A, and it's got the glucosinolates, which boost immune system and protect against oxidative damage (from the free rads that cause aging). Cabbage is also a cancer fighter (breast), and it's even been shown to defend against Alzheimer's disease. Green and red, cooked and raw: all good.

Garlic. You probably don't need much arm-twisting here; garlic automatically kicks cooking and eating up to the next level, and you'd probably have to use it even if it were really bad for you. Lucky thing, it's not. Garlic has great powers to protect against many types of cancer, including prostate, ovarian, breast, and colorectal. It's a fine source of vitamins C and B_6 and of protein, and of course it has basically no calories. Use it in cooking and marinades, and dressings and drizzle, and definitely on a daily basis.

Lettuce. Anything called greens is good. Not just lettuce lettuce (romaine, crisphead, butterhead, leaf), but the leafy things we like to think of as lettuce: radicchio, spinach, mustard greens, collard greens, watercress, arugula, kale, parsley. Remember when we talked about Americans eating so fast that our brains don't have time to send out the satiety signal? A smart salad is quick to stimulate that satiety hormone (called CCK) when eaten prior to the meal, and a bowl of mixed greens can give even an American eater a run for the money.

Onions. Huge anticancer capabilities: ovarian, prostate, breast, throat, mouth, and more. Also huge culinary capabilities. Onions make about anything you cook taste even better. Learn to use often. And don't forget to also make ample use of the onion's very respectable cousins: the scallions, shallots, chives, and leeks.

Soy. Because you decided you didn't like it even before you knew it was a vegetable? Okay, soy*beans*. You like beans, and these are a small miracle, both cheap and highly available (the United States is the world's largest producer). Soy products, such as edamame and tempeh, but with the possible exception of the candy bars, deliver big on protein, and have minerals to burn. Plus soy makes a good showing of potassium, calcium, and iron. Tofu, which is soybean curd, has long been championed for its youth-promoting properties, is said to help prevent bone loss in women, and has been proven to lower low-density lipoproteins (thus raising good cholesterol). Lately, questions have come up about tofu, as some studies show it raises estrogen in men as well as women; so don't overdo it until we hear something more definitive here. However, other, fermented soy products such as tempeh, miso, and soy sauce are still confidently recommended. Soy is also a fine source of fiber, with an enviably low GI. It's an inexpensive source of valuable protein, features plant-based omega-3s, and has been shown effective in preventing heart disease, osteoporosis, and cancer. Eaten regularly, it's an impressive all-round antiager.

Spinach. So they say, calorie for calorie, it's the most nutritious green thing on planet Earth. That's a very good reason to eat spinach *every day*. But if that alone is not enough to sway you, following are some of the herculean feats that regular spinach-eating is known to perform: helps prevent cancer, including skin, lung, stomach, colon, ovarian, prostate, breast; helps prevent stroke, cardiac, and artery diseases; helps your eyes; and improves cognitive decline. Here are a few of the reasons why: antioxidants, B, betaine, carotenoids, chlorophyll, coenzyme Q10, iron, vitamin K, minerals, plant-derived omega-3 fatty acids, polyphenols, calcium . . . Do you really need to hear the complete list? Just do as Grandma said and eat the spinach. Rumor has it there's no better vegetable in the world.

Sweet potato. It's a cash cow of nutrients and an absolute jackpot of vitamin A. The A comes in the form of carotene (hence the carrotlike color), which may help, if taken through whole foods and not supplements, to reduce risk of lung cancer. Good for the liver and anti-diabetes. A veg (and the only potato) known to stabilize blood sugar. That's a big one if you want to get and stay young, slim, and good-looking. You knew this moment was going to come: time to trade in the fries and the other tired old white ones for a colorful, magical, "hot" potato.

Tomatoes. You know this one, too; it's the alphabet: A, C, K, Bs, E, and more. Plus, the fire-engine red looks really good on your plate. Cooked tomatoes are rich in the antioxidant lyco-pene—a known cancer-preventer and/or retarder, notably pros-tate. And here's a bonus if you eat your broccoli: the benefits from the lycopene seem to increase when the two vegetables are eaten together—a nutritional double-header. If for no other reason, how could we cook, or eat, without the lovely tomato? They make even pizza and ketchup somewhat respectable. (Buy organic ketchup and tomato paste, though, because then the skin is included, and it's a big part of the important lycopene delivery system.) Eat cooked tomatoes often; it's the gentle cooking, in just a bit of olive oil, that releases the lycopene is such a way that it's readily bioavailable. With prepared tomato-based products, find ones low in added sugar, and of course free of HFCS.

Other excellent vegetables: arugula, asparagus, beets, carrots, cauliflower, celery, chard, collard greens, cukes, escarole, egg-plant, green beans, kale, mushrooms, okra, peppers, pumpkin, turnips, sprouts, squash, watercress, zucchini . . .

Beans and Legumes

High protein, *no cholesterol(!)*, and inexpensive, for starters. Black beans, white beans, kidney beans, red beans, fava beans, lentils, chickpeas. Great beans like these have long been either snubbed or neglected in the typical American diet. But all that's about to change as we learn more about this excellent food. A single source of the Big Three—good fat, good protein, and good fiber—beans are a complex carb that provide slow but steady energy to our muscles and nervous systems. They are rich in B vitamins and iron, are readily available, and—did we mention?—are a high protein source that *contains no cholesterol*. Another great thing to recommend beans is their usual low ranking on the Glycemic Index— but you should check the particular kind of bean on the list if you're trying to lose weight. They are good for our digestive systems, help lower bad cholesterol, and help fight cancers. Long a staple of Mediterranean and other heart-healthy international diets, beans taste delicious (and go easier on the digestive tract) when served with a drizzle of olive oil. They can be prepared or dressed with flavorful spices like antioxidant-rich oregano, rosemary, cilantro, fennel, turmeric, dill, lemongrass, or bay leaf—because, as we'll see, each of these has unsung-hero, youth-boosting powers, too.

Fruit

More plant food? Well, that's kind of the theme at first here. You can eat as many of the trace-level GI vegetables in as big portions as you like, and the more varieties you incorporate into every day and every meal, the better. On the other hand, fruit is a little more problematic if you want to lose weight. Why? Why else? . . . Because of the sugar. So if weight loss is your main objective, cut down on fruit at first (we'll make an exception with daily berries and an occasional apple or orange), avoid all fruit juices, and be selective. Once you're satisfied with the way you're losing weight, then start incorporating more whole fruits into your daily diet; they're too beautiful to lose. But avoid canned (the syrup), pre-served (the sugar), and fruit juice in place of the whole fruit. We know you know the phrase "an apple a day . . ."—which is as true as it ever was, and you appreciate the wondrous C-conveying qualities of your delicious orange—but here are a few other ex-traordinary fruits that should be eaten regularly for their amazing nutritional, medical, and beautifying capabilities:

Avocado. It's known as nutrient-packed because it's dense in C, E, K, B$_6$, folate, *and* it beats out the banana as a powerhouse of potassium. As a good source of healthy monounsaturated fat, from its considerable amount of oil (more so the rough-skinned Hass variety and less so the smooth-skinned Florida variety), the avocado helps to reduce bad blood cholesterol, raise good blood cholesterol, and satisfy appetite.

———

Artichokes. Don't waste your time wondering if it's in fact a fruit or a vegetable; you're going to need that time to eat it. While artichokes are not a showcase for any particular nutrient, they do deliver the goods, with a little bit of this and a little bit of that, which amounts to a food you don't want to miss out on, because it's better than a multivitamin. You don't have to eat artichokes every day, they're a bit exotic for that, but when you do, you'll get lovely levels of calcium, iron, niacin, phosphorus, magnesium, potassium, and vitamins A, C, and K. It's a low-calorie fruit, which makes it an ideal weight-loss food. And preparing and eating them is kind of a leisurely, elegant treat.

Blueberries. How hard can it be to remember to eat the only blue food . . . just about every single day? Tie a string around your finger—because this is exactly what we're going for—a food to be eaten often, completely on purpose, because it portends weight loss and youth-recovery in every beautiful blue bite. Blueberries are low in calories, sweet and delicious, chock-full of antioxidants, and eating them often will immediately start a wholesome process of skin repair. Look to them for some C and E, but especially for the phytonutrients, which help our cells fight free radicals and cancer (colorectal in particular), and of course skin aging. If you eat about a ½ cup to 1 cup of blueberries every day for the duration of the plan, you won't need convincing; you'll see it in the mirror. If you want to switch it up, take a blueberry break with blackberries. They are even higher in antioxidants and have a lot of luscious nutrients, including A, C, E, and lutein, which protects your eyes and may help prevent lung cancer. As a bonus, berries are high in fiber, so automatically slow down sugar conversion. Another plus is that they can be frozen without compromising the integrity of the nutrients, so are, in effect, available all year round.

———

Olives and olive oil. There is one fruit juice we want you to have on a daily basis: olive oil. You've heard a lot already about this celebrity food: but just to review. . . . This is a star source of the A+, monounsaturated fats you need to eat every day, and with which you'll replace other fats like trans fats (totally) and saturated fats (to a degree), thus becoming slimmer, better looking, and more heart-healthy. But if you can only remember one good reason to use this oil every day, remember your beating heart. Olives and the oil from the fruit protect from heart disease and high blood pressure, from stroke and breast cancer, and even wrinkles. Need we mention the iron, the E, the fiber, the lutein, and the beta-carotene? It would be hard to find a more perfect food for our purposes; if you do only one thing to get back your youth, inside and out, this is it. Buy extra-virgin, cold pressed. Use in dressings or drizzle, and be careful not to overheat when using for cooking, or you risk compromising the integrity of the nutrients. Canola oil has a higher smoke point, so if you tend to use high heat, keep it on hand or try a combo olive-canola oil, which is available in most supermarkets. (Another trick: coat the food in the oil before putting it in the pan, which will help control the oil's heat.) Take daily.

———

Pomegranates. Personally, I'm a little put out with the pomegranate craze, because pomegranate juice is a perfect example of how food processing reduces a perfectly wonderful fruit to a pile of sugar. But as for the pomegranate itself, you can see what all the excitement is about. The French named the hand grenade after the pomegranate for its scattershot seeds, but perhaps the potency of its nutrients would have been as good a reason. It's loaded with potassium, folic acid, C, and fiber. It's a no-nonsense antioxidant with strong phytochemicals and the famous polyphenols (some studies show even more than red wine), plus it's been shown to reduce risk for heart disease, to lower blood pressure, and to retard the progression of cancers. With all that at stake, it's worth the time and effort to get at the seeds. If you must drink the juice, seek out the one lowest in sugars and stick with that brand.

Other look-fabulous fruits: strawberries, blackberries, raspberries, cranberries, goji berries, grapes, apples and oranges, cherries, grapefruit, pears and peaches

Fish

Salmon. Two words: your skin. This delicious fish, the one even fish haters will admit doesn't taste half bad, has the omega-3 fatty acid dermatologists love because it renews the suppleness of the skin *and* protects against ultraviolet rays from the sun. This is exactly what we've been talking about: an accessible food that improves both health and beauty in one bite. Besides the omega-3s, this known "brain food" delivers D, a few good Bs, selenium, niacin, and of course protein. Eat often if you can buy wild; about once every third or fourth day if it's farmed. Canned is okay too, for salads or salmon burgers. Eating fish of any kind *just once a week* has been shown to protect against heart disease and to substantially lower risk of Alzheimer's disease. While on the youth-recovery plan (and then after the youth-recovery plan) increase the frequency with which you eat all fish, and especially wild salmon. (Note: Be a good student and monitor the debate about mercury levels in fish, and limit, but not necessarily eliminate, consumption of farm-raised fish.)

Other fine fish: cod, bass, wild tuna, sole, tilapia, lake trout, whitefish, mackerel, sardines, anchovies, and herring.

Meat

Grass-fed, organic beef. Because otherwise it's hard to know what you're having for dinner by way of antibiotics, hormones, and chemicals. All of the beautiful nutrients of beef—excellent iron, protein, B vitamins—are far more predominant (like ten to fifteen times more) in grass-fed as opposed to corn-fed cattle. Yes, beef is a source of saturated fat, but here's a little-known fact: half of the fat you eat with beef is monounsaturated (that's the good kind you get with olive oil). Yet there are real reasons, both health and beauty, to limit beef intake to far smaller portions than in the past (for one, iron is an oxidant; for two, there are as good or better sources of protein). Best health choice hands down is USDA-certified 100 percent organic. Best portion choice is about 4 to 6 ounces, which, if you're like most Americans, will probably weigh in at about half of what you were eating before.

Poultry

Turkey. Because every day could be Thanksgiving Day. The lowly turkey is a great source of lean protein, and vitamin B_3 helps stabilize blood sugar (and you now know what that means in terms of weight maintenance and damage control). The powerful antioxidant selenium in turkey helps thyroid and immune function. Also, turkey is economical and convenient (available already cooked in delis and in markets). Buying organic, free-range will ensure you won't be consuming antibiotics and hormones with your turkey dinner. Eat turkey at least once a week, not once a year; your body will bow its head and thank you for it.

———

Other good meats: lean pork, free-range chicken.

Nuts and Seeds

Almonds. Some heart specialists have bottom-lined it this way: you can eat almonds or you can take statins. The tasty and elegant little treasures have actually been shown to lower bad cholesterol *as effectively as drugs.* To most Americans who've spent years being indoctrinated against all fats, nuts are now one of those counterintuitive foods, the kind you have to relearn, the kind that fight fat *with* fat. Over 90 percent of the fat found in almonds is unsaturated fat, which we now know works to *lower* bad cholesterol. They are a fine protein source and offer fiber, calcium, magnesium, potassium, vitamin E, and the antioxidants and phytochemicals that are so good for you and your skin. Almonds also seem to have a special link with lowered risks of diabetes, Alzheimer's, and cancer.

Walnuts. They're small but they're powerful. Eating a handful of walnuts as a midday snack or before a meal, on a regular basis, several times a week, can significantly reduce risk of heart disease, diabetes, and cancer—the very diseases that American health statistics are plagued by. Now that we know more about good fats, we can start to enjoy good nuts; indeed, the omega-3s in walnuts decrease the risk of cardiovascular disease and increase arterial health. Like almonds, walnuts contain healthy protein and fiber. Eat often (but not too many at a time) if you want to lose weight.

Other great nuts and seeds: cashews, pistachios, peanuts, hazelnuts, pecans, sunflower, hemp, flax, pumpkin

Dairy

Yogurt. You know the drill. Don't buy the tricked-out, show-pony yogurt featured floor to ceiling in your supermarket, because it's chock-full of sugars. Buy plain, full-fat, or low-fat (but not no-fat) yogurt and add the berries or other fruits or nuts, add the spices (a little cinnamon or nutmeg?) yourself, and if you want sweetness, a dash of certified organic agave natural sweetener (available at health food stores), or a packet of raw sugar or some molasses or organic honey: all good, and good enough for you in moderation. Some of the reasons to go out of your way to eat yogurt include: it has more calcium than milk does; and it has vitamin B, phosphorous, and healthy bacteria from fermentation. Plus, not to get overdramatic about it, but it decreases risk of no less than death. It is a brilliant antiager that protects against infection and inflammation, and as a bonus it's said to increase female fertility. Greek yogurt, though slightly more expensive, is highly recommended, as it delivers the highest protein, with about 11 grams per serving. Eat yogurt daily.

———

Cheese. We've made a point so far of shunning packaged foods labeled *low fat*, *fat free*, or *no fat*. And for good reason: these processed foods often contain trans fats, sugars, and other additives. But as far as the low-fat dictum, cheese (and maybe yogurt) may serve as the exception to the rule. It's not that full-fat cheese is bad for you—in moderation, if you don't need to watch your weight, and if you get enough of the A+ Fats that help to break down cholesterol. And we far prefer the natural selections at the cheese shop to the often processed selections in the dairy section of the supermarket. But some cheeses that have reduced fats—cheese from skim or partly skim milk—are fine. Part-skim mozzarella (for melting), natural feta (for salads), and reduced-fat hard cheeses (for snacks) can be used sparingly while you're controlling weight. Parmigiano-Reggiano is a classic with fantastic flavor, and since we don't tend to eat too much of it, it gets a free pass for shaving on top of your vegetables or salad. It's worth remembering that as a rule, hard cheeses are higher in protein and lower in fat than creamy cheeses such as blue, goat, Brie, etc.

————

Other good dairy: eggs, kefir, milk, cottage cheese

Grains

Barley. For the fiber. Also for its excellent track record at reducing blood sugar. It's an anti-inflammatory that can lower the bad cholesterol. You can mix it into rice, salads, or stews, have it in soups, or find a bread that features it.

————

Oats. Oats have been proven to lower cholesterol *better than drugs*, even more so if you're eating oat bran. Both are a great source of fiber and are packed with nutrients. Many studies have shown that regular consumption appears to substantially lower risk of heart disease. Oats make for delicious bread, and thick, steel-cut oatmeal makes a great basic breakfast that you can adorn with all sorts of other List foods. Always start with whole, slow-cooking oats, not instant, because with fiber, as we know, slow is what it's all about.

————

Other good grains: buckwheat, millet, quinoa, brown rice, bulgur, wheat germ, wild rice

Spices and Herbs

Turmeric. This tasty spice is a triple-threat antioxidant, anti-inflammatory, and antimicrobial food. It contains great iron, fiber, potassium—and it's been studied for its suspected role in preventing cognitive decline, like that associated with Alzheimer's disease. If it sounds exotic, it's really not; it's related to the ginger plant and is often found in curry powders and mustards.

———

Oregano. For such a little flake, this is an impressive antioxidant. It's positively loaded with antiaging capabilities, has a whole alphabet soup of vitamins and minerals, has been known since ancient times to guard against infection, and has been proven more effective than drugs at treating some bacterial diseases. Besides, where else can you get 2 teaspoons of pure flavor for less than 10 calories? Add it to your tomato and other sauces even if it's in there already; more is better.

———

Rosemary. It not only has a memorable flavor, it's said to increase memory and focus, as it fortifies brain cells against free rads. It's also a known cancer fighter and detoxifier. To help protect against carcinogens from charring, add it to your burger on the grill or to steak in the pan. If you learn to use this native Mediterranean herb absolutely all the time, you will only increase the flavor of most meats and vegetables while decreasing the chances of cognitive decline.

Honey and Chocolate

We don't want to force these on you while you're on a "diet," but both are pretty good for you if you don't overdo it. With honey, you can make your own energy or sports drink, or use a teaspoon to sweeten your morning yogurt or oatmeal, or afternoon tea. Though its GI is on the high side, and it's not a particularly outstanding source of nutrients, natural honey has the skin-boosting polyphenols that your dermatologist will surely appreciate—and besides, if you're looking for a little sweet, it's a better choice than refined sugar, and certainly better than HFCS.

———

As for chocolate, you've heard the buzz; the cocoa component in chocolate is rich in minerals, including copper, magnesium, potassium, and manganese. You get phytochemicals, another form of antioxidant, here, too. Dark chocolate (forget the milk chocolate or even drinking milk with chocolate, and we're sorry that includes chocolate ice cream; the milk appears to negate the benefits) is an impressive all-round antioxidant, and that's good for reversing aging of the skin and other fine things. Best of all, the cocoa phenols in dark chocolate can help lower blood pressure. The higher the cocoa content, the better, so look for chocolate around the 70 percent mark, or the highest you can go without finding it more bitter than sweet.

———

Other age-proofing and health-promoting herbs and spices: Well, it's come to pass: we can't pick a winner. The fact is, all herbs and spices are great for you, and learning to use them often and consistently in cooking will impart untold health and beauty benefits—each spice in its own special way. Herbs and spices are rich in life-extending flavonoids, cell-rebooting antioxidants, and cancer-defeating anti-inflammatories. These all help to youth-recover you fast. Find ways to regularly include the ones mentioned above as well as sage, tarragon, parsley, basil, marjoram, thyme, black pepper, cayenne pepper, cinnamon, ginger, coriander, yellow curry powder, cumin, cloves, allspice, apple pie spice, nutmeg, mustard, anise, dill, Aegean sage, fennel, mint, savory, sea fennel, sumac. All of them will do something for you long- and short-term.

Drinks

Coffee. Besides the fact that most of us love it and refuse to live without it, brewed coffee's got good fiber. Who knew? Studies by Spanish researchers show your cup of Joe has a decent amount of the kind of soluble fiber (dissolves in water) that helps fight bad cholesterol and prevent heart disease. Studies also show that coffee helps prevent Parkinson's disease in men, breast cancer in older women, and diabetes in younger women. These impressive studies, however, were not done on vanilla lattes or dolce cappuccinos or any similarly over-the-top coffee drinks, aka desserts now sold by the billions everywhere from coffee shops to coffee emporiums to fast-food franchises. Avoid any flavoring syrups in your coffee. They are loaded with sugars. And of course, don't douse it with sugar yourself. A little milk or half-and-half won't hurt you, but unfortunately, we don't know if we can say the same for artificial sweeteners. The word is still out here, and it doesn't look good for aspartame and the other pretenders. But since you no longer get way too much artificial sweetening in diet soda and other diet drinks, maybe it's okay to use substitutes sparingly. Saccharin has been around the longest and some studies show it's the safest. We would probably prefer USDA-certified organic agave nectar, for its admirable GI rating (though here again, not too much). Also, buy organic coffee if you can, as there are mounting concerns over how pesticides are used in growing beans.

————

Tea. It's a warm and cozy—or a cold and refreshing—sip of smart medicine. The medicinal qualities of various teas have been suspected for centuries, but lately, studies have proven a specific benefit for regular tea drinkers against cardiac illnesses and heart attack and against prostate and other cancers. The key health ingredient in tea is the catechins in the leaves—a category of flavonoids, which is a category of antioxidant. Dermatologists love tea for the skin repair and protection potential, particularly when it's flavored with lemon—a combination that's been shown to protect against skin cancer. Black, white, and green teas are all good for antiaging. The only issue with tea seems to be that to get the benefits, you have to drink quite a lot of it. Many of the studies that showed significant impact for tea drinkers on diseases ranging from cancers to rheumatoid arthritis were done on people drinking four to ten cups a day. But probably less is still better than none. Since it's a treat with no carbs, no fat, and no calories, it can't hurt to make it a habit. It may be an acquired taste, but learn to drink it straight, with lemon, and all right, maybe a little honey; over time, it could have surprising health and beauty benefits.

————

Wine. Does living long while feeling sublime sound good? That seems to be what the excellent antioxidant resveratrol in wine—I'm duty bound to add "in moderation"—can do for you. If you're a wine lover, you've already been heartened to hear of its health-inducing properties: a big reduction in risk of heart disease and stroke, anticancer capabilities, increased good cholesterol, reduced stress, and of course it makes good food even better. Drink wine with a proper meal featuring protein, because that helps make the resveratrol bioavailable. Best never to drink wine or any alcohol on an empty stomach anyway—it'll bypass your heart and go straight to your head and make you stupid. Although white wine has resveratrol, too, red has more. But, despite the TV ads, grape juice really doesn't cut it. It's the fermentation in wine that gives it its special powers. Recommended daily limitation is one to two glasses for women, two to three for men. If you don't drink alcohol, try taking a good-quality resveratrol supplement, available at vitamin stores.

Water. It's the best and only real way to quench thirst; it fills up your stomach so makes you less hungry, is good for your skin, transports nutrients around your system, disposes of toxins, and tastes terrific. Drink flat, tap, sparkling but always without added anything—unless it's an ice cube or a squeeze of fresh lemon. Drink it a lot, with meals and in between. Filter it at home, carry it around in a lightweight, lined, long-lasting, good-looking, ecofriendly water bottle (about $20 at most sporting goods stores), and try like anything to cut down on your consumption of plastic. Many plastic bottles have been shown to leach chemicals into the bottled water that weren't there to start with, rendering it far less "pure" than advertised, and of course their proliferation is a huge issue for our environment. (To get a sense of scale on this, I recommend the eye-opening and engaging *Bottlemania* by Elizabeth Royte.)

The Meals

By now you know that the new world of weight loss and/or youth-recovery is meant to be easily organic—meaning you take in the knowledge, make the adjustments little by little, and the results happen, quite effortlessly.

So you don't really need someone standing over you saying what you should eat for each meal. You can follow the recipes offered, or you can branch out on your own. Here comes the fusion part, where we apply what we now know about food history and science and culture to buying, preparing, and eating. But first a few reminders:

Let's Review . . .

Plants. Make meals of mostly plants and plant-based foods. Animal protein is fine if you're not opposed to it, but for the reasons discussed should be cut down to size. Eat more fish and less red meat, and look for other, good, nonanimal protein sources—don't be shy and try some soy, or some strange new, low-GI bean. Cook with A+ Fat, which is plant-based fat; don't forget, this is how you fight fat with fat. Be especially indulgent with leafy greens, and insist on seeing color on your plate like never before. Good color is a good sign that you're getting the variety of nutrients, and all the beautiful antioxidants, that protect health and recover youth.

———

Water and wine. Drink plenty of water. Most likely: more than before. H_2O is good for us, and it helps fill us up so we don't feel hungry for the wrong kinds of food. Beer (maltose: one of the fastest sugars) is out if you're losing weight, but limited wine is allowed. If your main purpose is to shed pounds, don't drink wine until you've seen some satisfying weight loss, and then reintroduce it sparingly.

———

Tea and coffee. All sodas and sugared energy drinks are banned—whether or not you need to lose weight. Coffee and tea are fine. A little milk or honey is allowed, and so is a little sweetener, as advised, if it means that much to you.

———

Spices. Antioxidant-rich spices are encouraged. Almost all spices and herbs are very, very good for you, each in its own particular way. They will also help prime your skin for instant and effortless self-renewal mode.

———

Snacks. Between meal minifeedings are necessary. As we discussed, hunger does not help you lose weight; in fact, it hurts. Nuts are a good way to regularly get the fat that's famous for satiating and keeping your appetite under control. (Just take care to eat a handful, not a family-size jar.) Processed snacks, as we now know, do the opposite—increase your appetite, along with the glycemic load—and so no matter how cute and harmless they sound, must be given the heave-ho.

———

True Food, slow food, and *new* food. We were told that one reason this approach to daily diet worked well for our patients is because it gradually expanded, and permanently altered, their "world" of food. We had suggested that they experiment with foods they had ignored before, if only to get them in the mood for change. So if you want the same results, you are honor-bound to try new food as well. Make a little thing of meeting at least one new food daily: a food you've never had before, or something maybe you tasted once but dismissed, or like but routinely forget to eat. Try this every day for thirty days. You won't be close to done with all the great food in the world by reunion day. Maybe today it's a new spice. Maybe today it's a different sort of vegetable, like a sweet potato instead of the same old, same old white potato. Maybe today is a double day: the day you cut up some tempeh and cook it with vegetables a new way in a new kind of pan. Try a new fish with a funny name, a low-GI grain so foreign it's borderline intimidating, a bean you honestly never laid eyes on before. Ask what it is at the market, buy it, look up a recipe for it, cook it, eat it. Just order it, if you must. This practice alone will give you a fresh new perspective on daily diet, and a whole new lifestyle that sticks.

The Plan

This isn't one of "those" diets, so we're not going to spoon-feed you strict menus that you probably won't follow for more than a day or two anyway. Besides, telling you exactly what to eat is counterproductive—and a good way to kill not only your appetite but your new NIQ.

Still, some people like a little guidance in the kitchen, so we've come to a kind of compromise. It works like this:

Breakfast. We'll itemize seven sample breakfasts, which you can change or repeat, week by week. These were suggested by our fitness expert, Kacy Duke, a wonderfully strong and lithe woman whom we can only imagine leaps out of bed each glorious morning ready to greet the new day. Some of the recipes are the same ones she recommends for her sensationally fit movie star clients when she's training them for their death-defying action sequences in major motion pictures. You'll find them detailed in *The Magnificent Seven*.

———

Lunch. For lunch, you're on your own. All we'll do is list some delicious possibilities—meaning if you listen to us, you'll be eating a salad. At least it will resemble a salad in that it's built on fresh greens, but it will also deliver the good fats we're so fond of, and the protein you can't live without. Of course, you don't have to eat a salad for lunch to quickly lose weight and/or look great. If you have the luxury of time (and money), you can steam a lobster and some asparagus, drizzle on some tarragon vinaigrette and a squeeze of fresh lemon, and ask the butler to please serve you poolside. Or, if you're one of those ladies who lunch, you're in luck. True Food is easy to get in a great restaurant. But practically speaking, most of us are eating lunch at home or at our desks most days. One of the easiest prepared foods to find near the office is a salad, replete with a tasty portion of protein and a lavish assortment of plants. The names of the salads on the lunch list will tell you everything you need to know to find an approximation of them ready made, or to make them at home. Experimentation is encouraged, as long as the ingredients are all True Foods. In honor of our ancient ancestors, these lunch suggestions are grouped under the heading *Hunt Your Lunch*.

Dinner. The big question of the day, of every day, is, of course, What's for dinner? True, we could have walked down the hall and asked the no-nonsense nutritionist the very question. But as knowledgeable as she is, and as skilled at dishing out the tough love to clients who need to lose twenty-five pounds or more, we feared if we gave her the opportunity, she'd have us all living on naked lettuce and bare chicken. So we had another idea. Who better to ask what's for dinner than some of the people who had cooked themselves dinners every night based on HSR-recommended foods and had slimmed down and looked great as a result? We asked some of our patients. (I told you we're into fusion.) Of course, the patients we asked were the ones who were already accomplished home or pro cooks to begin with. Patient-doctor privilege prevents us from revealing their names, but we do have permission to give a sound bite on their stories.

Mark

"Mark," still a great athlete way into his forties, injured his knee playing basketball at the gym, and while recovering from surgery, gained fifteen pounds. He adopted a diet of True Food and lost twenty. He's an excellent cook who hustles up dinner for eight with the speed of a power forward, and some of his favorite main courses are featured here.

Jill

"Jill," a former professional ballerina and a famous entertainer, had found it hard to keep off the pounds after hip replacement surgery. She, too, took on True Food, now serves it up to her guests, and receives the same adulation as ever.

Daniel

"Daniel," a major talent on Wall Street, lost his job in the dustup after the recession hit in 2009. He gained weight and got depressed, though he's not sure in what order. He's since switched to the right food, lost twelve pounds, and has started a small but successful consulting firm.

A few things these HSR dieters all have in common: they all trimmed down, shaped up, feel and look younger and better than ever. And, they can cook.

The recipes our guest chefs recommended were for main courses they had devised or adapted to suit True Food parameters: made of fresh ingredients, heavy on The List foods, and a dish they liked well enough to use as a staple and to recommend to you. Their suggested dinner entrees are found in the section *Our True Food*.

You'll also get a list of Snacks and a list of Sides. Snacks can be taken midmorning and midafternoon, and don't hesitate to have a few nuts or another good-fat food a few minutes before dinner, to help appease your appetite. The Sides are all recommended plants, so you can choose two, three, or as many as you like, to grace your main course. The more variety of the recommended plants you can start consuming on a daily basis the better; each of the featured foods has something very special to offer the youth-recovery effort. Once you try these combinations and the preparations, and see the results in your looks and energy level, we suspect you'll want to make HSR eating a way of life.

The Code Again

Level One: weight loss and youth-recovery combined. You'll stick to the most basic preparations and the lower glycemic foods until you've lost the first five to ten pounds, and have a head start on permanent weight control. If there's a note indicating Level Two next to a food offered on a recipe, then don't eat it until around week three, or when you're satisfied with your initial weight loss. After that, you can begin to introduce Level Two foods.

Level Two: better looks, better health, and younger skin. At this level, you don't need to lose more than a couple of pounds, most likely at your waist. You can eat suggested fruits, whole grains, nonwhite rice, even whole-wheat pasta, and have wine with meals.

Whether you're Level One or Two, remember we've *all* already given up trans fats, HFCS, processed foods with high sugar content, no-fat-labeled foods, instant and fast foods, and of course too much dessert. If you're Level One and you need to lose weight, you'll have to do a little more to step up your game, and take the first few weeks to get into training. For you, the new diet will initially be a bit more rigorous. Don't worry, that part will go quickly and be painless because you'll be eating healthy fats to control hunger and curb appetite. You'll get to eat as much as you want of certain foods, but the following ones are to be avoided until you've mastered True Food.

Avoid the following foods on Level One:

- Most fruit and fruit juices, for now (free pass on daily berries, and an occasional apple, orange, or grapefruit)
- All but one serving of whole-grain bread, for now
- All boxed cereals
- All pasta
- All rice
- Corn and potatoes, except an occasional sweet potato
- Carrots, peas, beets, and any high-GI veg or legumes
- Veal, duck, sweetened ham, and any fatty cuts of meat
- Cheese (except for very moderate Parmesan, feta, goat, and cottage)
- Ice cream and other desserts
- Soda, including diet, for good (and good riddance)
- Beer and the hard stuff
- Wine, for now, except in cooking

Menu Plans

7-Day Level One Meal Plans

If a significant part of your HSR diet plan is moderate weight loss, chances are, you need a few days to detox from the stealth sugars you've been getting too many of in one form or another. An initial week to ten days of detox will stabilize your blood sugar and keep your appetite under control—which is the one sure way to achieve lasting (and, fast, and effortless) command over your weight.

If you did your homework, you know by now what to eat: smart carbs, good fiber, A+ Fats, and great proteins. You know to pay attention to the Glycemic Index rating of foods—even fruits and vegetables—always, but especially during the phase when you want to lose pounds quickly to start the permanent weight control process. You know to make a daily habit of nutrient-rich, unprocessed True Food, and to ditch anything that doesn't fall into the category.

This is all by way of saying that you don't need to follow specific daily meal plans, because you now *have* the tools. You *know* what to do. But if you're the type who prefers training wheels when learning to ride a bicycle—or maybe the type who hasn't ridden a bicycle in absolute years, or the type who just likes to be told, chop chop, then here you go: seven sample days. You can change it as you see fit. And feel free to pile on as many low-glycemic vegetables as you want, lunch and dinner, to your heart's content.

Day 1

Breakfast

- Magnificent Seven 1: Green Eggs and Ham (page 154)
- Water, coffee, or tea, with a splash of milk or squeeze of lemon

AM Snack

- 1–2 slices organic turkey

Lunch

- Grilled chicken, arugula, and sesame seed salad with Dijon mustard vinaigrette
- Water, flat or sparkling

PM Snack

- 8–10 walnuts, ½ an apple
- Tea: green, black, or white

Dinner

- Pan-seared Sea Scallops with Balsamic Reduction (page 191)
- Steamed or oven-roasted asparagus spears (served with a drizzle of olive oil) (page 194)
- Mixed greens salad with chopped vegetables (i.e., red or green or yellow peppers, cucumbers, tomatoes, onions); 1–2 tablespoons olive-oil-based vinaigrette
- ½ cup blueberries or strawberries with one packet of raw sugar or ½ teaspoon organic honey
- Water, flat or sparkling; decaffeinated coffee or tea

Day 2

Breakfast

- Magnificent Seven 7: Beauty in a Blender, Level One (page 161)
- Water, coffee, or tea, with a splash of milk or squeeze of lemon

AM Snack

- Cherry tomatoes and ½ cup cottage cheese

Lunch

- Fresh or canned tuna and mixed lettuce salad with dill and white wine vinaigrette
- Water, flat or sparkling

PM Snack

- 12 raw almonds
- Tea: green, black, or white

Dinner

- Baked free-range chicken breast with assorted fresh herbs and lemon
- Sauteed fresh spinach and pine nuts (page 194)
- Mixed greens salad with chopped vegetables (red or green or yellow peppers, cucumbers, tomatoes, onions); 1–2 tablespoons olive-oil-based vinaigrette
- Water, flat or sparkling; decaffeinated coffee or tea

Day 3

Breakfast

- Magnificent Seven 5: Kacy's Westside Egg White Omelet (page 159)
- Water, coffee, or tea, with a splash of milk or squeeze of lemon

AM Snack

- ½ cup plain yogurt, sweetened with ½ teaspoon of agave and ½ cup blueberries

Lunch

- Goat cheese, walnuts, and cherry tomatoes on mixed greens with red wine and thyme vinaigrette
- Water, flat or sparkling

PM Snack

- 2 celery sticks stuffed with natural peanut butter or cottage cheese
- Tea: green, black, or white

Dinner

- Salmon with Wine and Fresh Rosemary (page 170)
- Broccoli or cauliflower roasted with garlic (page 196)
- Mixed greens salad with chopped vegetables (red or green or yellow peppers, cucumbers, tomatoes, onions); 1–2 tablespoons olive-oil-based vinaigrette
- Water, flat or sparkling; decaffeinated coffee or tea

Day 4

Breakfast

- Magnificent Seven 6: Oatmeal with Brown Sugar on Top (page 160)
- Water, coffee, or tea, with a splash of milk or squeeze of lemon

AM Snack

- ½ cup of pistachios

Lunch

- Turkey "club" salad with smoked turkey and cherry tomatoes on baby spinach with lemon-tarragon vinaigrette
- Water, flat or sparkling

PM Snack

- Hummus and raw vegetables
- Tea: green, black, or white

Dinner

- Tilapia South of the Border (page 171)
- Steamed green beans with a drizzle of olive oil
- Mixed greens salad with chopped vegetables (red or green or yellow peppers, cucumbers, tomatoes, onions); 1–2 tablespoons olive-oil-based vinaigrette
- ½ cup of fresh mixed berries with ½ teaspoon of agave or organic honey, sprinkled with cinnamon
- Water, flat or sparkling; decaffeinated coffee or tea

Day 5

Breakfast

- Magnificent Seven 2: Sweet and Spicy Triberry Yogurt (page 155)
- Water, coffee, or tea, with a splash of milk or squeeze of lemon

AM Snack

- Whole apple

Lunch

- Smoked salmon, red onion, and tomatoes on mixed greens with balsamic vinaigrette
- Water, flat or sparkling

PM Snack

- 12 raw almonds
- Tea: green, black, or white

Dinner

- Seared Sirloin with Spice Rub (page 187)
- Roasted sweet potato (page 195)
- Sauteed spinach with garlic cloves
- Mixed greens salad with chopped vegetables (red or green or yellow peppers, cucumbers, tomatoes, onions); 1–2 tablespoons olive-oil-based vinaigrette
- Water, flat or sparkling; decaffeinated coffee or tea

Day 6

Breakfast

- Magnificent Seven 4: Citrus Classic (page 158)
- Water, coffee, or tea, with a splash of milk or squeeze of lemon

AM Snack

- 1 cup of plain yogurt sweetened with ½ teaspoon of agave or organic honey, with ½ cup blueberries or strawberries

Lunch

- Greek salad: kalamata olives, cucumber, and crumbled feta cheese on red leaf lettuce with garlic-lemon red wine vinaigrette
- Water, flat or sparkling

PM Snack

- Small bag of sunflower seeds
- Tea: Green, black, or white

Dinner

- Simple Salmon with a Kick (page 176)
- Basil Broiled Tomatoes (page 198)
- Steamed broccoli with a drizzle of olive oil
- Mixed greens salad with chopped vegetables (red or green or yellow peppers, cucumbers, tomatoes, onions); 1–2 tablespoons olive-oil-based vinaigrette
- Water, flat or sparkling; decaffeinated coffee or tea

Day 7

Breakfast

- Magnificent Seven 3: Fiesta Frittata (page 156)
- Water, coffee, or tea, with a splash of milk or squeeze of lemon

AM Snack

- Orange

Lunch

- Niçoise salad: fresh or canned tuna, niçoise olives, green beans, and anchovies on mixed greens with red wine vinaigrette
- Water, flat or sparkling

PM Snack

- 12 raw almonds
- Tea: green, black, or white

Dinner

- Fresh Herb-Roasted Chicken (page 179)
- Steamed spinach with a drizzle of olive oil
- Baked onions with thyme
- Mixed greens salad with chopped vegetables (red or green or yellow peppers, cucumbers, tomatoes, onions); 1–2 tablespoons olive-oil-based vinaigrette
- Water, flat or sparkling; decaffeinated coffee or tea

Breakfasts

The Magnificent Seven

Green Eggs and Ham

Sweet and Spicy Triberry Yogurt

Fiesta Frittata

Citrus Classic

Kacy's Westside Egg White Omelet

Oatmeal with Brown Sugar on Top

Beauty in a Blender

Breakfast 1
Green Eggs and Ham

Scrambled eggs, or poached, if you please, prepared with something glo-riously green: sautéed spinach, steamed asparagus, diced green peppers, finely chopped broccoli or Brussels sprouts, parsley, watercress, chives, chervil, or anything else green and edible you've got. Level Two can add a slice or two per person of Canadian bacon (leaner than the American kind). If the kids are included, a dash of green food coloring (organic of course) helps them take the dish literally, so they learn their lessons well. The gist of it is to get them (and you) accustomed to green as a color at breakfast. This recipe is for scrambled eggs with spinach, though you're encouraged to try Green Eggs and Ham every which way you can.

Serves 1

    1 to 2 cups fresh spinach
    2 eggs
    1 or 2 tablespoons olive oil (cold pressed, virgin)
    Coarse salt, ground pepper
    Canadian bacon, 1 or 2 pieces (Level Two)

Rinse the spinach and cook with the water remaining on the leaves over high heat in a skillet until spinach wilts. Remove to a bowl.

Whisk eggs with a tablespoon of water, preferably with a wire whisk (helps fluff), preferably in a copper bowl (also helps fluff).

Heat the olive oil in the skillet, add the eggs, and stir with a fork until partially cooked. Add the spinach, salt, and pepper and cook to de-sired doneness. Meanwhile, brown the Canadian bacon in a skillet and serve it with the green eggs. (Level Two can add a slice of whole-wheat toast with butter.)

Breakfast 2
Sweet and Spicy Triberry Yogurt

Berries are one of those foods to eat every day because they're a beauty food, full of skin-promoting antioxidants. The dash of cayenne pepper is great for glowing skin, and helps healthy digestion. Berries are virtually available all year round because they freeze well, and they're relatively inexpensive as a staple. They're actually not negotiable on the thirty-day plan, because lots of berries, particularly blueberries, are essential to priming the skin for full youth-recovery. So get used to eating a cup or even more of berries every day—though Level One should limit consumption to about half a cup while losing weight.

Serves 1

1½ cups plain or Greek yogurt
Sweetener of choice: 1 teaspoon of agave, raw honey, grade B
    maple syrup, or a sprinkling of raw (not refined) sugar
Dash of cayenne pepper
6 to 10 raw almonds or walnuts
¼ cup raspberries or strawberries
¼ cup blueberries
¼ cup blackberries

Combine the Greek yogurt, sweetener, and cayenne pepper. Toss in the nuts. Fold your red and blueberries into your white yogurt, salute the colors, and enjoy!

_____ **Breakfast 3** _____
Fiesta Frittata

Another way to get your AM protein and vegetables, but with a little gratis international flair, a frittata offers a fresh approach to breakfast-as-usual with a splash of style. You can serve this one with salsa (home-made is best; if you use store-bought, of course first check the label for sugar). You can throw in a little—but not too much—cheese (reduced fat is okay for Level One). The distinction of the frittata is that extra egg whites are added, and it's either flipped over (here a frittata pan helps), or it's cooked partially on the stove and then in the oven. Easy as pie; far better for you.

For a festive occasion, this one serves 4.

2 to 3 tablespoons extra virgin olive oil

¼ cup sliced green onions

½ cup chopped red bell pepper

3 tablespoons chopped jalapeño

2 small plum tomatoes, diced

2 tablespoons fresh chopped basil or 1 teaspoon dried

4 eggs

4 egg whites

Salt and freshly ground black pepper

¼ cup sharp or extra-sharp grated Cheddar cheese

Heat the oven to 350 degrees F. Heat the oil in a 10-inch cast-iron skillet. Add the onions, red bell pepper, and jalapeño and sauté over medium heat for 3 minutes. Add tomatoes and basil and cook for 3 minutes or until tender. Whisk together eggs, egg whites, salt and pepper, then pour into skillet and cook over moderate heat until almost set, 3 to 5 minutes. Sprinkle cheese evenly on top, transfer skillet to oven and bake 5 minutes. Cut into triangular wedges. Level One: serve with ½ cup of berries. Level Two can have 1 cup of berries and buttered whole-wheat toast.

Variations on the Theme

Part of the beauty of the frittata is that it allows for so many exquisite combinations. Try to remember to make full use of the recommended look-good spices and fresh vegetables. For example, you can combine these:

Turkey bacon and rosemary
Mushrooms and chives, tarragon, chervil
Arugula and shallots
Bermuda onions and smoked salmon
Sweet onions and fresh oregano
Asparagus, goat cheese, and proscuitto (Level Two)

It's a blank canvas for culinary inventiveness, and the result is always easy on the eyes.

Breakfast 4
Citrus Classic

What could put one more in mind of sunrise at ocean side? . . . The classic half grapefruit gets a little raw sugar or a drizzle of honey or real maple syrup on top—plus a heap of blueberries to make the plate pop.

Level Two, you can serve it with a slice or two of whole-wheat or other whole-grain toast. (Good idea: you need the toast to transport the fat that's in the butter to your mouth.)

Level One, keep it to one slice of whole wheat and, in place of butter for now, a teaspoon of natural peanut or almond butter, which have benefits beyond just taste. Or in place of the grapefruit, substitute a whole orange, the kind you sit there and leisurely peel.

Serve with the sound of rolling surf and the morning paper.

Serves 1

1 grapefruit or orange
1 to 2 pieces whole-wheat toast
Butter or natural peanut or almond butter

Breakfast 5

Kacy's Westside Egg White Omelet

This delicious omelet is a twist on the traditional French version show-casing egg whites, sans yolks. Filled with sautéed spinach, mushrooms, and onions, it's full of protein and the skin-boosting, everyday antioxidants vitamins C and E.

Serves 2

2 tablespoons light olive oil
1 cup prewashed baby spinach
½ small onion, diced
¼ cup small baby mushrooms, sliced
6 egg whites
¼ cup milk
Salt and freshly ground black pepper to taste
Nonstick cooking spray
Parsley sprig, for garnish (optional)

In a nonstick pan with the olive oil, sauté vegetables together or one at a time until desired doneness. Remove as much moisture as possible from the spinach and set the vegetables aside. In a small bowl, whisk together the egg whites, milk, and salt and pepper. Spray the pan, preheat it over medium heat, then add the egg mixture. Stir and then reduce heat to medium-low. Let egg mixture cook until firm. (Cooking the eggs at a low temperature will ensure a soft, fluffy omelet.)

Remove from heat and top with sautéed vegetables. Fold the omelet in half, slide it onto a plate, and garnish with a sprig of parsley for presentation's sake.

Arty Tip: If you prefer your eggs yellow, adding a dash of turmeric will provide color and antioxidant power, too.

Breakfast 6
Oatmeal with Brown Sugar on Top

The cooking instructions for whole, slow-cooked, steel-cut oatmeal—the search-and-destroy replacement for processed breakfast cereals—usually requires about twenty to thirty minutes simmering time. Make it worth the wait by turning your bowl of oats into a treat. Add fat to this fiber-fest with a pat of butter (Level One) or a splash of milk (Level Two), add some antioxidant power with a sprinkling of cinnamon, and some protein punch with nuts, walnuts, almonds, or pecans. Feel free to appease your sweet tooth by tossing in a few slices of unpeeled apple and then drop a little brown sugar on top. Measure and cook oats according to instructions on the box or tin. Serves as many as you have.

———

Like most of the other breakfasts on the Magnificent Seven menu, the oatmeal itself only acts as the foundation, and you supply the real architecture by adding key nutrients and structuring the dish to represent all major food groups: carbs, protein, and fat. Eating this way first thing in the day will ultimately make you slimmer, not fatter. Any of these breakfasts is a much safer bet for weight and beauty control than not eating breakfast at all.

Breakfast 7

Beauty in a Blender

The smoothie or milk shake is unfailingly fresh and feel-good for the breakfast on the run. It's another blank canvas, and you supply the artistry: maybe adding a little soy or hemp powder, or flaxseed oil. Here we added açaí (ah-sah-ee), which is a fruit from Brazil with an exotic berry flavor and the natural synergy of antioxidants, essential omegas, amino acids, and fiber—making it one of nature's most powerful antioxidants. Below are two versions, for Levels Two or One.

Beauty in a Blender, Level Two

Serves 1 (Level Two)

1 pack Sambazon brand frozen pure unsweetened açaí (found in
    frozen-fruit section)
½ cup frozen mixed berries
1 banana
1 cup coconut water
A scoop of whey protein powder, for an extra boost

Mix everything together in the blender until smooth. This creamy, rich shake is a great skin treatment, and a healthy start to the day.

Beauty in a Blender, Level One

Here's a smoothie alternative, with a lower glycemic count. It's also an opportunity to get creative and add nutrient-rich spices: sprinkle nutmeg or cinnamon on top, add a drop of pure vanilla and a teaspoon of honey, and garnish with a slice of citrus.

Serves 1 (Level One)

½ cup milk (skim is okay)
½ cup plain yogurt
½ cup frozen strawberries
½ cup frozen blueberries
1 teaspoon honey
4 ice cubes

Mix everything but the ice together in the blender until smooth. Add the ice and puree again until rich, creamy, and perfectly chilled.

Lunches

Hunt Your Lunch

Here are some salads we all can enjoy. Meat or fish portions should be limited to less than 4 ounces. Vinaigrette is generally made with 2 parts oil to 1 part vinegar. For those on Level One, if a recipe calls for nuts or cheese, use them very moderately; keep it to six or eight nuts, and a shaving or single crumbling of cheese. And limit oil to 1 to 2 tablespoons to dress the salad on your 9-inch plate.

- Endive, artichoke hearts, and proscuitto salad with lemon-mustard vinaigrette
- Niçoise salad: tuna, green beans, niçoise olives, and anchovies on mixed greens with red wine vinaigrette
- Goat cheese, walnuts, and tomatoes on red and green leaf lettuce with red wine and thyme vinaigrette
- Frisée and Belgian endive with toasted pine nuts and pomegranate seeds and red or white wine vinaigrette
- Grilled chicken, arugula, and sesame seed salad with Dijon mustard vinaigrette

163

- Fresh tuna and mixed lettuce salad with dill and white wine vinaigrette
- Spinach salad with toasted pecan halves and Dijon mustard vinaigrette
- Curried chicken and diced apples served on mixed greens with sweet mustard vinaigrette
- Radicchio, arugula, and boiled egg salad with red wine and oregano vinaigrette
- Red and green oak leaf lettuce with grated Gruyère and Dijon mustard vinaigrette
- Shrimp and shallots served on butter lettuce with fresh dill and lemon vinaigrette
- Greek salad: kalamata olives, cucumber, and crumbled feta cheese on red leaf lettuce with garlic-lemon-red-wine vinaigrette
- Romaine lettuce, boiled egg, and Parmesan salad with anchovy Caesar vinaigrette
- Endive, walnut, and apple salad with lemon vinaigrette
- Smoked salmon, red onion, and tomatoes on mixed greens with balsamic vinaigrette
- Boiled shrimp, cherry tomatoes, and spring onions on Boston lettuce with lemon, garlic, and Dijon vinaigrette
- Grilled tempeh served on radicchio with tahini (sesame) lemon vinaigrette
- Lump crabmeat, tomatoes, and baby romaine salad with lemon-tarragon vinaigrette

- Steamed lobster salad: cold, cut-up lobster on a bed of mixed greens with lemon-soy vinaigrette
- Turkey "club" salad: baby spinach, smoked turkey, and cherry tomatoes with lemon-tarragon vinaigrette

Snacks

- Cottage cheese (½ cup) and cherry tomatoes
- Olives (8–10)
- Nuts: walnuts, almonds, pistachios (1½ to 2 ounces)
- Seeds: pumpkin, sesame, sunflower (small bag, approximately 2 ounces)
- Kefir on low-GI granola (¼ cup)
- Canned salmon or tuna (1 can)
- Celery sticks spread with natural peanut or almond butter (2 sticks)
- Turkey breast (2–3 ounces)
- Yogurt (6 to 8 ounces) with berries (½ to 1 cup)
- Pear or apple with a small piece of hard cheese
- Hummus and raw vegetables, cut up

And, for late nite fans of Chelsea Handler and her sidekick Chuy (pronounced "Chewy") . . .

- The Chelsea Chuy: Celery sticks with organic almond butter or organic peanut butter and a drizzle of organic honey.

- The Chuy Chelsea (Level Two): Medley of red, green and/or black grapes. Mix with a handful of (unsalted) almonds, pecans and/or walnuts.

Dinners

Our True Food

Salmon with Wine and Fresh Rosemary

Tilapia South of the Border

Asian Flank Steak

Pork Chops with Crushed Fennel and Garlic

"Not-Your-Mama's" Tuna Casserole

Simple Salmon with a Kick

Broiled Swordfish with Lemons and Capers

Lamb Chops with Fresh Tarragon and Shallots

Fresh Herb-Roasted Chicken

Sautéed Sea Scallops in Shallot Sauce

Shrimp Scampi

Spiced Indian Chicken

Whole-Wheat Pasta with Tuscan Herbs

Seared Sirloin with Spice Rub

Sautéed Shrimp with Asparagus and Brown Rice

New York Minute Dinner Salad

Grilled Lamb Chops with Rosemary and Lemon

Pan-Seared Sea Scallops with Balsamic Reduction

Salmon with Wine and Fresh Rosemary

The idea is to make a point of eating as many of the recommended foods in as many ways on as many days as possible—and still have something surprisingly dishy to please you at every meal. This extremely simple and quick fish can be made as well with fresh fennel—just sub the fennel for the rosemary and serve up a completely different taste.

Serves 4

2 pounds salmon, with the skin
1 teaspoon sesame oil mixed with 1 teaspoon olive oil
2½ cups white wine or part wine, part water
A generous handful of fresh rosemary from the garden or the
    farmer's market, leaves removed, some sprigs reserved
Coarse salt and freshly ground pepper

Cut the salmon into four individual servings and rub with the oil mixture. In a large skillet over medium-high heat, bring the wine to a boil and reduce the liquid by half. Reduce heat to low, add the rosemary leaves and the salmon. Simmer covered for 5 to 8 minutes, until fish is firm and done to taste. Season with salt and pepper, and serve garnished with the reserved sprigs of fresh rosemary.

Tilapia South of the Border

These are widely available fish fillets that can be prepared a number of inventive ways. A good opportunity to use lively spices and benefit from their healing powers while indulging a bit of exotic taste.

Serves 4

2 cups chopped cilantro
3 tablespoons olive oil
1 tablespoon chopped chipotles in adobo
1 tablespoon water
1 teaspoon ground cumin
Coarse kosher salt
Freshly ground black pepper
4 tilapia fillets, about 4 ounces each

Preheat the broiler.

In a blender, combine the cilantro, olive oil, chilies, water, cumin, salt, and pepper, and puree until the sauce is smooth.

Place the fish in a pan lined with foil and add the pureed sauce. Broil fish until cooked to preferred doneness, from 7 to 10 minutes.

Asian Flank Steak

The soy-based marinade gives an appealing Asian kick to this easiest of grill steaks. Get in the habit of adding soy sauce and/or rosemary or other herbs and spices to grilled or broiled meat—or to sprinkling some onto your al dente cooked vegetables. These flavor enhancers add good health as well as pleasingly exotic taste. But before you buy: even soy sauce has to be checked for sugar or HFCS content; read the label or buy organic if you can.

Serves 4–6

¾ cup soy sauce
½ cup olive oil, plus more for brushing
3 tablespoons organic honey
6 to 8 garlic cloves, minced
3 to 4 tablespoons chopped fresh rosemary
1 teaspoon dried rosemary
1½ tablespoons coarsely ground black pepper
2 teaspoons coarse kosher salt
2-pound flank steak
1 bunch of grilled scallions, for serving

Make the marinade by mixing all the ingredients except the scallions and steak. Pour it over the meat; cover and refrigerate for 1 to 2 hours. Remove the meat from the marinade and grill the steak over medium-high heat for about 5 minutes per side. Brush the scallions with oil and grill them alongside the steak. While the steak is setting, arrange the scallions around the edge of the platter. Slice steak across grain and serve in center of platter.

Variations on the Theme

- Try a mixture of ¼ cup soy, fresh grated ginger, and sesame oil (1 teaspoon) on tilapia fillets, then grill.

- Brush a mixture of ¼ cup soy, ¼ white wine, a squeeze of fresh lemon juice, and Dijon mustard (2 teaspoons) on salmon fillets and roast or grill.

- Or try ¼ cup soy and a dash of sesame oil on sirloin steak before grilling.

Pork Chops with Crushed Fennel and Garlic

An inventive yet simple way to make spices and herbs part of every day.

Serves 4

2½ teaspoons coarse kosher salt

3 teaspoons crushed dried fennel

1 teaspoon finely chopped fresh flat-leaf parsley

1 teaspoon freshly ground black pepper

4 1½- to 2-inch-thick bone-in pork rib chops

Pour of olive oil

5 garlic cloves, minced

½ cup white wine

1 cup chicken broth

In a small bowl, mix 2 teaspoons of the coarse salt, the fennel, parsley, and pepper; rub the mixture all over the chops. Let stand for about an hour or refrigerate, covered overnight. In a heavy skillet over medium heat, thinly cover the bottom of the pan with and heat the olive oil. Add the chops and sear, about 4 minutes per side. Transfer the chops to a plate. Pour off all but 3 tablespoons of the drippings and olive oil from the skillet. Add the garlic and sauté for 1 minute. Add the wine, then broth, and bring to a boil. Return the chops to the skillet, reduce heat to low, and simmer covered until thoroughly cooked yet tender, about 140 degrees internal temperature.

"Not-Your-Mama's" Tuna Casserole

The new age of cooking fresh and in season is a far cry from the old tuna casserole recipe with the optional potato chip topping found on the back of the mushroom soup can. But you don't have to lose the casserole dish. Several A-list foods are found in this main course—garlic, onions, and tomatoes, olive oil and fish, plus a little resveratrol-rich wine. Still easy and still feeds a crowd.

Serves 6–8

3 tablespoons olive oil
2 large onions, peeled and sliced thin
2 pounds tuna steaks, cut into servings
Coarse salt and freshly ground black pepper
2 heads of garlic cloves, peeled and halved
2 pounds fresh tomatoes, peeled, seeded, and chopped coarse
2 cups red wine
3 bay leaves
3 tablespoons chopped parsley, plus leaves for garnish

Heat the olive oil in a heavy-duty casserole dish; add the onions and cook over low heat, covered, until tender and translucent, about 5 minutes. Remove the onions, turn heat to high, and sear the tuna in the remaining oil, just 1 to 2 minutes per side. Remove tuna from heat and sprinkle with salt and pepper.

Add the onions, garlic, tomatoes, wine, bay leaves, and parsley back to the casserole dish with the tuna and simmer over low heat for 1 hour. Sprinkle with fresh chopped parsley and serve.

Simple Salmon with a Kick

You don't have to go the casserole route. This extremely simple and quick fish can be made with tuna as well.

Serves 4

Here's the Kick
　　2 thumbs of ginger, grated with a grater or zester
　　1 tablespoon wine vinegar
　　1 tablespoon soy sauce
　　1 teaspoon toasted sesame oil
　　1 tablespoon mirin

　　2 pounds salmon, with the skin
　　2 pounds spinach, washed
　　1 tablespoon canola oil

Whisk together all the "kick" ingredients. Let the mixture sit while you prepare the rest.

Steam the spinach and set it aside.

Heat the canola oil to hot in a skillet, then very quickly sear both sides of the salmon, about 2 to 4 minutes per side, depending on your preference for doneness.

Arrange spinach on a platter or split among individual plates, place salmon on top, then drizzle with the kick ingredients.

Broiled Swordfish with Lemons and Capers

Easy and elegant, swordfish is an excellent way to eat fish and still have "a steak."

Serves 2

4 garlic cloves, peeled and minced
Olive oil
2 tablespoons capers
1 fresh lemon in wedges, plus 1 lemon sliced thin
Coarse salt and freshly ground black pepper
2 swordfish steaks, about 4 ounces each
Fresh parsley, for serving

Crush the garlic with a mortar and pestle, and drizzle in a tablespoon or two of olive oil. Mash in the capers and squeeze the juice from 2 or 3 lemon wedges into the mix. Season liberally with salt and pepper.

Brush the swordfish on both sides with a little olive oil. Broil the steaks for about 2 minutes per side, or cook to taste. (Also great on the grill.)

Top with the caper sauce and serve with the lemon slices and parsley.

Lamb Chops with Fresh Tarragon and Shallots

A sophisticated way to make a flavor-filled main course in less than 20 minutes.

Serves 4

4 1¾-inch-thick lamb chops
Coarse salt and freshly ground black pepper
Olive oil or butter (Level Two)
3 tablespoons shallots, finely chopped
2 heaping tablespoons fresh, chopped tarragon or 1 tablespoon
   dried

Season the chops with the salt and pepper. Broil them about 4 inches from the flame, about 7 minutes per side. Remove to a serving platter.

Melt 3 tablespoons of butter (Level Two) or olive oil (Level One) in a saucepan over low heat and add the shallots and tarragon. Cook for 2 minutes, remove from heat, and drizzle over the chops.

Fresh Herb-Roasted Chicken

Here is the reward for shopping fresh at the farmer's market: a succulent chick infused with flavor. Note how easily the eat-every-day spices can make a simple dish special. You can experiment with the herbs: use tarragon and thyme, marjoram, rosemary, parsley, or sage—they make it almost impossible not to create a masterpiece of a home-cooked meal.

Serves 4 to 6

Coarse salt and freshly ground black pepper
1 4 to 5 pound roasting chicken, free range if available
Butter or olive oil
1 or 2 garlic cloves, peeled and sliced (optional)
Half a lemon
½ cup white wine
¼ cup fresh thyme, chopped
¼ cup flat-leaf parsley, chopped
3 tablespoons tarragon, chopped
1 large onion, sliced
2 celery stalks, sliced
2 carrots, grated
1½ cups chicken stock

Hours ahead, salt and pepper the chicken, including the skin and cavity, and refrigerate. To prepare: Preheat oven to 400 degrees F. Rub the chicken with butter (Level Two) or olive oil (Level One) and, if using garlic, place the slices between the skin and the flesh. Place the half lemon in the cavity. Truss the legs with kitchen twine and place the chicken on a roasting rack in a roasting pan.

Cook the chicken in the middle of the preheated oven for half an hour, then add the wine and the herbs and vegetables to the roasting pan. Reduce heat to 350 degrees F and continue roasting, basting often with the pan juices, for about another hour and 15 minutes, until juices run clear from the thigh when pierced with a knife. If the top of the chicken begins to turn too brown, cover it loosely with foil. When the bird is done, transfer it to a platter.

Pour off the fat from the roasting pan, and place the pan (with the cooked herbs, vegetables, and any juices) on the stove over medium-high heat. Add the chicken stock and cook, stirring, for about 5 minutes. Strain the sauce and serve it over the chicken with additional freshly ground pepper.

Sautéed Sea Scallops in Shallot Sauce

This dish delivers maximum dazzle for minimum effort, especially if you shop smart and buy premade fish stock from the local fish store. The seared scallops taste and look delightful on a plate with sautéed spinach and/or broccoli rabe, garnished with a lemon wedge.

Serves 2

1 cup fish stock
2 tablespoons shallots, peeled and minced
2 garlic cloves, peeled and minced
1 tablespoon fresh rosemary, minced
2 lemon wedges, plus more for garnish
⅓ cup olive oil, plus a little more for searing
1 pound large sea scallops
Coarse salt
Ground pepper

Place the fish stock in a small saucepan over medium heat and reduce the amount to a little less than half.

Mix the shallots with the garlic, rosemary, and the juice from the lemon wedges. Whisk in the reduced fish stock and the olive oil, combining thoroughly.

Heat 1 to 2 tablespoons olive oil in a skillet over medium heat. Season the scallops with salt and pepper, add them to the skillet, and cook them for about 5 minutes, turning once, until golden brown. Serve drizzled with the shallot sauce and garnished with lemon.

Shrimp Scampi

Shrimp is a crowd-pleaser, and this dish is simple and flavor filled. But because of the fairly high butter content, it's only for Level Two. Even then, don't make a habit of it; but you already know better.

Serves 4

6 tablespoons (¾ stick) unsalted butter, at room temperature
¼ cup olive oil
1 tablespoon minced garlic
1 tablespoon minced shallots
2 tablespoons snipped fresh chives
Coarse salt and freshly ground black pepper to taste
¼ teaspoon paprika
2 pounds large shrimp, peeled and deveined

Preheat the broiler.

In a large bowl, combine the butter, olive oil, garlic, shallots, chives, salt and pepper, and paprika. Blend thoroughly. Add the shrimp to the mixture, thoroughly coat it and place in a broiler pan.

Broil the shrimp close to the flame for 2 minutes on each side. Serve immediately.

Spiced Indian Chicken

This dish is infused with the aromatic spices that do so much to beautify your skin.

Serve with plain yogurt topped with diced apples and a dash of cinnamon.

Serves 4

Marinade
   ¼ cup olive oil
   ½ cup chopped onion
   2 garlic cloves, minced
   1 tablespoon fresh chopped ginger or ¼ teaspoon dried ground
   ½ teaspoon ground cumin
   ½ teaspoon curry powder
   ¼ teaspoon ground turmeric
   ¼ teaspoon cayenne
   Pinch of ground cinnamon
   Pinch of ground nutmeg
   Pinch of red pepper flakes, rubbed between fingers
   1 tablespoon white wine vinegar
   4 skinless and boneless chicken breast halves
   Coarse salt and freshly ground black pepper
   1 to 2 tablespoons olive oil
   ½ cup chicken broth

Mix together all the marinade ingredients in a glass bowl. Add the chicken breasts, coat thoroughly, cover, and refrigerate for 3 hours to overnight.

To prepare, remove chicken breasts from the marinade and pat them dry. Season with salt and pepper. Heat the olive oil over medium-high heat in a heavy skillet. Add the chicken breasts and sauté until golden brown, 2 to 3 minutes on each side. Add the chicken broth and the marinade to the skillet and bring the liquid to a boil. Reduce heat to low and simmer for 6 to 8 minutes, stirring occasionally, until the chicken is done. Serve with yogurt and apples for Level One, and add a cup of steamed brown rice for Level Two.

Whole-Wheat Pasta
with Tuscan Herbs

A Level Two special treat, this simple main-course pasta is bursting with Mediterranean flavor and fresh, antioxidant-rich herbs.

Serves 4

1 pound whole-wheat pasta (spaghetti or penne)
Dash of salt

For the Sauce

4 tablespoons olive oil
2 garlic cloves, finely chopped
8 anchovy fillets in oil, drained and chopped
2 tablespoons canned tomato puree
2 to 3 tablespoons finely chopped fresh
    flat-leaf parsley
1 tablespoon each finely chopped fresh thyme,
    rosemary, and marjoram
Crushed dried chilies
Salt and freshly ground black pepper
Fresh grated Parmesan cheese (optional)

To cook pasta: Bring a large saucepan of salted water to a boil, add the pasta, add a drop of oil, and cook for 7 to 11 minutes, until al dente (tender, but not overcooked).

To prepare the sauce: Heat the olive oil in a small saucepan. Sauté the finely chopped garlic until it just begins to change color. Transfer the olive oil to a skillet, reserving the garlic in a separate container. Add the chopped anchovies to the skillet and cook over very low heat, stirring until they dissolve into a smooth paste. Stir in the tomato puree and cook for 1 minute. Add the chopped herbs and stir over low heat for 2 minutes. Add the reserved garlic and remove the pan from the heat.

Drain the pasta and put it in a large deep bowl. Pour the sauce over the pasta and toss well. Add the dried chilies, and salt and pepper to taste. Top with grated Parmesan cheese.

Seared Sirloin with Spice Rub

Raise the antioxidant quotient a notch by getting inventive with spices for your sautéed steak.

Serves 4

1 teaspoon dried oregano
½ teaspoon five-spice powder
½ teaspoon sweet paprika
½ teaspoon salt
¼ teaspoon pepper
1 pound boneless sirloin steak
2 garlic cloves, finely minced
2 teaspoons canola oil
2 teaspoons olive oil

To make the spice rub: In a small bowl, stir together the oregano, five-spice powder, paprika, salt, and pepper.

Coat the sirloin evenly on all sides with the spice mixture. Set the meat on a plate for 10 minutes. Heat canola oil in a heavy skillet over medium-high heat and sear the steak for 5 minutes on each side for medium-rare. Transfer to a plate. Pour the fat and oil out of the skillet, then add 1 to 2 teaspoons of olive oil and the garlic; cook it over medium heat for about 1 minute, until the garlic is gold. Return the meat to the pan and cook for 2 minutes. Slice and top with the warmed pan sauce.

Sautéed Shrimp with Asparagus and Brown Rice

Here's a quick shrimp dish without butter, and the wholesome addition of brown rice (for Level Two). Level One, serve with a fresh greens salad and vinaigrette dressing with a splash of lemon.

Serves 1

1 tablespoon light olive oil
½ cup sliced asparagus
1 small tomato, diced
Salt and freshly ground black pepper to taste
5 or 6 fresh large or jumbo shrimp (cleaned and deveined)
Cayenne pepper (optional)
1 or 2 scallions, sliced
½ cup of brown rice (Level Two)

Heat the olive oil in a medium sauté pan over medium heat. Add the asparagus and sauté it for 4 to 5 minutes. Add the diced tomato and season with salt and pepper; cook another 3 minutes.

Season the shrimp with salt, pepper, and cayenne pepper, if desired.

Add the shrimp to the pan and reduce the heat to medium-low; cook for 5 minutes.

Top the shrimp with the sliced scallions and serve over brown rice or with a salad of fresh greens.

New York Minute Dinner Salad

This colorful salad incorporates canned tuna as well as fresh vegetables and is a light, quick, and delicious way to eat dinner and get out the door.

Serves 2

1 bag prewashed mixed greens of choice
1½ bell peppers, thinly sliced (use a combination of red, yellow, or
    orange peppers)
¼ cup fresh flat-leaf parsley
2 small or 1 medium-size tomato, sliced
1 small red onion or 2 scallions, sliced (optional)
2 6-ounce cans tuna in olive oil
1 teaspoon balsamic vinegar
Salt and freshly ground black pepper to taste

Combine all vegetables in a large bowl and top with the tuna. Mix and season with balsamic vinegar, salt, and pepper.

Grilled Lamb Chops
with Rosemary and Lemon

When craving a meat-based meal, turn to savory lamb chops to satisfy taste without weighing you down.

Serves 4

4 1¾-inch-thick lamb chops
Salt and freshly ground black pepper to taste
1 tablespoon extra-virgin olive oil
1 teaspoon freshly squeezed lemon juice
1 teaspoon rosemary, dried or fresh
4 lemon wedges

In a large bowl, season the lamb chops with the salt, pepper, olive oil, lemon juice, and rosemary.

On a stovetop grill or in a sauté pan over medium heat, cook the chops for about 4 to 5 minutes per side or until desired doneness.

Top the lamb chops with pan juices and garnish them with lemon wedge.

Pan-Seared Sea Scallops
with Balsamic Reduction

Another supremely simple take on the scallop, this one works well for both levels.

Serves 1

¼ cup balsamic vinegar
4 sea scallops (2 to 3 ounces each)
Salt and freshly ground black pepper to taste
1 tablespoon extra virgin olive oil
1 cup mixed greens

In a small saucepan over low heat, heat the balsamic vinegar until it reaches a syrupy consistency. Keep it warm.

Season the scallops with salt and pepper. Heat the olive oil in a small sauté pan and add the scallops. Cook them over moderately high heat until each side is seared and caramelized, about 1 to 3 minutes on each side, or until cooked through.

Cover a plate with mixed greens and arrange the scallops on top. Drizzle with the balsamic reduction.

Sides

You'll find that in the following suggested side dishes, we haven't gone all specific about the exact amounts to buy and serve. This is a good place to develop your natural eye for proportion, and thus enhance your skills as a cook. Choose amounts according to how many people you'll serve: with a portion being what would look about right on the plate. Would you eat about six Brussels sprouts? Then if you're serving two people, buy about twelve. You can judge most vegetable amounts just by looking, and logic: one artichoke per person; one sweet potato; a healthy handful of green beans each. Watch out for spinach, though; it's notorious for shrinking down during cooking. Buy more than you think you'll need—about 8 to 10 ounces per person (though spinach lovers have been known to dine on a pound). Otherwise, try out your eye for size; it's an important part of your nutritional evolution. If you make a mistake you'll be an expert the next time.

Sautéed Fresh Spinach and Pine Nuts

Heat olive oil over low heat in a skillet; add 1 or 2 minced garlic cloves and about 1 tablespoon of pine nuts per serving. Cook for 1 to 2 minutes, until the garlic and nuts brown. Then add about half a pound of spinach per person. Sauté on medium-high, stirring, until the spinach wilts, about 3 minutes. Season with salt and pepper.

Green Beans Tossed with Walnuts

Parboil the green beans (about ¼ pound per person) in boiling water until al dente, about 3–4 minutes. Sauté about 1 teaspoon chopped walnuts per serving in a skillet over medium-high heat with a little butter or olive oil and a dash of walnut oil for about a minute. Add the beans and continue to sauté for about 3 minutes. Serve with salt and pepper.

Oven-Roasted Asparagus Spears

Snap off the tough ends of the asparagus spears, place the spears on a baking sheet, and drizzle them with olive oil. Roast in a 450-degree oven for about 10 minutes. Serve with salt, pepper, a squeeze of fresh lemon, and maybe a dusting of fresh-grated Parmesan.

Wine-Braised Red Cabbage

Core and slice a head of red cabbage into strips. Place it in a heavy oven-proof saucepan with a little olive oil, a cup of red wine, a cup of chopped onion, ⅓ cup of balsamic vinegar, and salt and pepper. Bring to a boil on the stove, then cover and cook in a 350-degree oven until tender, about an hour.

Oven-Roasted Brussels Sprouts

Trim the bottoms of the Brussels sprouts. Liberally coat them with olive oil and season with salt and pepper. Place in a shallow roasting pan and cook for about 30 to 40 minutes in a 400-degree oven. Serve with salt, pepper, and a little chopped parsley.

Roasted Sweet Potato

Coat a whole sweet potato with olive oil, season with salt and pepper, and roast in a 400-degree oven until done, about 40 minutes. To test for doneness, stick a fork in the potato, and see if it's tender yet still a little resistant to the touch. Cut it in half lengthwise and dress with a pat of butter (Level Two), or drizzle with olive oil. Liberally season with freshly ground black pepper, kosher salt, and the "special topping" of your choice: chopped rosemary, toasted sesame seeds, Parmesan, honey, ginger, orange zest, lime . . .

Pan-Sautéed Mushrooms, Sans Butter

Remove stems from your favorite mushrooms and wipe clean; leave the mushrooms whole or slice if you like. Heat a heavy saucepan or skillet over medium heat, add the mushrooms, and keep stirring. They will squeak as they seal in the juices and flavor and cook to perfection all by themselves—without butter or oil.

Broccoli or Cauliflower Roasted with Garlic

Parboil the broccoli or cauliflower florets for about 2 minutes. Sauté a clove or two of minced garlic in a few tablespoons of olive oil. Drizzle the oil over the florets, arrange on a baking sheet, sprinkle on salt, and roast for about 15 minutes in a hot (400 to 450 degrees) oven. Serve with parsley and pepper.

Steamed Artichokes

Remove the tough outer leaves and cut off all but 1 inch of the stem. Trim the hard tips of the leaves with scissors. Rub the entire artichoke with a fresh lemon, to prevent discoloration during cooking. Drop the 'chokes into boiling water, add some coriander seeds and a little lemon juice, and simmer covered for about 40 minutes. Serve with a basic vinaigrette of olive oil, vinegar, and Dijon mustard.

Baked Eggplant with Anchovy Sauce Parmesan

Combine 2 to 3 tablespoons olive oil, 1 tablespoon lemon juice, a clove or two of minced garlic, and 1 to 2 tablespoons anchovy paste; mix until blended. Slice 1 peeled eggplant into ½-inch rounds, coat them with the mixture, place on a baking sheet sprayed with cooking spray, and bake for 15 minutes in a 400-degree oven. Top with freshly grated Parmesan and freshly ground black pepper.

Sautéed Escarole

Trim off the stem end of each head of escarole. Wash well, then shake off the water. Heat olive oil over medium-low heat in a large saucepan, add 1 or 2 cloves minced garlic, cook briefly, and add the escarole. Cover and cook for 10 to 15 minutes. Sprinkle with salt, pepper, and maybe a little balsamic or white wine vinegar.

Braised Leeks

Trim off the tops and roots of the leeks. Cut the stalks lengthwise and hold under running water, washing leaves thoroughly. Heat a tablespoon of olive oil and a little butter over low heat in a skillet, and sauté one minced onion. Add leeks, about a cup of chicken stock (for 4–6 leeks) and some salt and pepper, and simmer for about 15 minutes, until tender.

Sautéed Marinated Mushrooms

Marinate cleaned, sliced mushrooms in olive oil, then pour off most of the marinade. Sauté the mushrooms over medium-high heat with some minced garlic and minced shallots for about 5 minutes. Serve with salt and pepper.

Green Beans and Pepper with Basil

Heat some olive oil over medium-high heat in a heavy skillet, then sauté some chopped onion, minced garlic, and a diced green pepper. Cook until the onions and peppers are softened; add a few tablespoons of water per pound of beans and a handful of chopped basil. Add about 1 pound of trimmed green beans; cover and simmer until tender, about 12 minutes. Top with salt and freshly ground black pepper and maybe a little Parmesan cheese.

Baked Onions with Thyme

Wash and dry one medium Bermuda or Spanish onion per person, sprinkle with dried or fresh thyme, and bake in the oven for about 1½ hours at 375 degrees. Remove the onions from the oven, cut off the root end, and peel off the skin. Serve with salt and pepper, and maybe a pat of butter.

Basil Broiled Tomatoes

Halve the tomatoes and drain them cut side down in a colander. Mix some olive oil, a handful of chopped fresh basil, salt, and pepper. Place the tomatoes in a heatproof baking dish, drizzle with the basil sauce, and broil for about 10 minutes. Top with chopped parsley and a little grated Parmesan.

Zucchini with Sliced Almonds

Sauté ½ tablespoon sliced almonds per person in a skillet with a little olive oil until lightly browned; then remove the almonds and set them aside. Cut one medium zucchini per person into thin slices, discarding the ends. Add a little more olive oil to the skillet and cook the zucchini with some minced garlic for about 3 minutes. Serve with the sliced almonds and maybe a little freshly grated Parmesan.

Sliced Brussels Sprouts with Sesame Seeds

Trim the Brussels sprouts, cut them lengthwise and slice very thin. Heat olive oil in a skillet over high heat and stir in the sprouts, some minced garlic, and a handful of sesame seeds. Add a little white wine and cook for about 3 to 5 minutes while stirring. Reduce heat and cook until the leaves are tender, add salt and pepper, and serve.

How to Lose Five Pounds in One Minute

Sorry, we forgot to tell you this. You could have lost five pounds in a minute if we'd remembered. Oh, well, better late than never. . . .

Standing and walking properly instantly makes you thinner, or at least makes it look like you are. From an MD's point of view, good posture means healthy alignment of the musculoskeletal system, so that joints, muscles, ligaments, and bones all pull their weight. It also keeps important organs (brain, liver) in position so they can function their little hearts out. You can't even be truly happy slouching because C-minus standing or sitting adversely affects the nervous system. And style-wise, for reunion day, no little black dress or new blue shirt can compete with the head-turning power of entering the gym walking upright. Even before you look your very best in the flesh, now is the time to get to a full-length mirror and study how you stand and walk.

See that your shoulders are level and parallel to the floor. Turn sideways and check that your head neither juts forward (too geezer) nor rolls back (too fat-guy). See that your shoulder blades are pulled down but relaxed, that your head and hips don't tilt to one side or the other, that your ankles turn neither in nor out, and that your arms and hands fall gracefully along the seams of your pants. Now try walking the walk, gently bending your knees so your butt doesn't shoot out too far behind and ruin the whole effect. Over the next few weeks, stand and walk and sit consciously until good posture becomes second nature. You'll look better, younger, slimmer, hotter—instantly.

C Ester and What You Just Did for Your Brain

Remember how one of the first things we recommended on the Cheat Sheet was that you take a daily **vitamin C ester**? You *do* remember . . . because you've been taking a daily **vitamin C ester.** You've doubtless already heard about the wondrous effect vitamin C has on the skin. So you probably figured C ester was first on our list because it can stimulate the rejuvenation of your skin via antioxidants and collagen renewal. Maybe we even threw that it's a good way you could keep from getting a cold. All true, but new studies show vitamin C may help our motor control as well. See, there's a part of our brain, the *nucleus accumbens*, that's key to movement, and it has a high level of natural C, but the level depletes over the years. And unlike other species, we humans can't produce our own C. We must rely on nutrition. Regular vitamin C is essential to life, and the **vitamin C ester** goes it one further because it is fat-soluble (penetrates cells better), has greater staying power at lower doses, and stands up better to oxidative stress. This is an example of another small adjustment in diet that resonates large over life. Oh, and did we forget to mention memory? The *hippocampus* in the brain needs a steady dose of C, too. See? All parts of the body, and the program, are key players on your medical dream team.

Endnote

School's out. On your own initiative, you've improved blood profiles, lost weight, gained knowledge, recovered youth, and "glamorized" skin texture and tone.

Dude!

See you at the reunion.

Acknowledgments

Thank you to the incomparable Jonathan Karp and the dream team at Simon & Schuster: our excellent editor, Kate Ankofski, publicity chief Victoria Meyer, publicity director Brian Ulicky, and associate publisher Aileen Boyle. Thank you to our ace publicists and good friends, Sandi Mendelson and Jennifer Fisherman Ruff; our eminent agent, Janis Donnaud; and our wonderful counsel, Eric Rayman, Esquire.

It is difficult to express enough appreciation for the support offered on a daily basis by the staff of the exceptional New York Dermatology Group. Thanks in particular must go to our terrific CEO, "JP" Van Laere, and to my talented fellow physicians: dermatologists Shilesh Iyen, MD, and Neha Parikh, MD, and internist John Adams, MD, for their uniquely modern take on skin health and internal medicine. Many thanks to Bahar Malekzadeh, MD, for her contributions to the NYDG medical and operational team. Great thanks and affection to fitness-expert-to-the-stars Kacy Duke; she has been an inspiration throughout the development of this project, and has brought her unique experience to bear on the finished product. We also thank her son, Milan Pizzacarola Duke, an aspiring professional chef in New

York City, for his expert contribution to the meals. Thanks to Shanna Honkomp for her keen editorial eye and depth of nutritional knowledge, and to Mark Rangle for his beautiful (and bright) cover design. Thank you to the entire "special" floor staff of NYDG for the input and the wit: Nancy Fonseca, Diana Morales, Kevin Yeroushalmi, Mariluz Felix, Natanya Massey—and the "guys": IT It-Boy Carlos Hernandez, shutterbug Christian Galan, and comic-in-residence Christopher Ryan. Many thanks to the lovely Kim Webb and the fourth-floor staff, and to our dear friend and colleague Kim Sevy. We love and appreciate both sisters Lisa (Reed for reading; Colbert for volunteering as first derm patient at seven years old), Mark Colbert—creative editor and surf partner—Leslie Reed, and Deb Zdobinski. Daniel Lucas and Kevin McCabe of Nimble Fitness, and power training couple Anthony and Lauren Dragos, thanks for teaching insights into health you don't learn in med school. Thirteen-year-old Charles Homans and twelve-year-old Harry Seabrook, you taught us something precious about True Food. Thanks to City Bakery for many a delicious, healthy fresh-market meal while writing this diet, and to master chef Anita Jacobson for her generous lessons in the art of cooking. And to Marianne Gillow, MD, Jerry Jodice, and Jeri Lee Jodice, thanks for the deeply appreciated contribution to the development of this book. Thank you all.

Recommended Reading

You didn't think you were getting out of here without your reading assignments. . . . Here are a few of the excellent books we've been inspired by, and we think you will be, too.

Pollan, Michael. *In Defense of Food*. New York: Penguin Press, 2008.

Royte, Elizabeth. *Bottlemania*. New York: Bloomsbury, 2008.

Schlosser, Eric. *Fast Food Nation*. Boston: Houghton Mifflin, 2001.

Read anything you can by the above three. Also highly recommended:

Agaston, Arthur, MD. *The South Beach Diet*. Emmaus, Penn.: Rodale Books, 2003.

Bittman, Mark. *Food Matters*. New York: Simon & Schuster, 2008.

Campbell, T. Colin and Thomas M. *The China Study*. Dallas: BenBella Books, 2006.

de Grey, PhD, Aubrey, and Michael Rae. *Ending Aging*. New York: St. Martin's Press, 2007.

Duke, Kacy, and Selene Yeager. *The SHOW IT LOVE Workout*. New York: McGraw-Hill, 2007.

La Puma, John, MD. *Chef MD's Big Book of Culinary Medicine*. New York: Crown, 2008.

Pollan, Michael. *The Omnivore's Dilemma*. New York: Penguin Press, 2006.

Roizen, Michael, MD, and Mehmet Oz, MD. *You: The Owner's Manual*. New York: HarperCollins, 2005. As seen on *Oprah*, all of the Roizen/Oz books deliver a wealth of medical information. Also recommended, for weight loss, their *You: On a Diet, Revised and Updated*. New York: Free Press, 2010.

Royte, Elizabeth. *Garbage Land*. New York: Little, Brown, 2005.

Taubes, Gary. *Good Calories, Bad Calories*. New York: Knopf, 2007.

———

We also recommend WebMD.com, one of the smartest and most accessible medical resources anywhere, available 24/7 on your computer screen. You can ask them anything and receive state-of-the-art answers from top medical specialists. Or click on "Food and Recipes" under Health A–Z. For skin care advice, you can search for Colbert at the site's Healthy Skin TV. And for a thorough reference on modern dermatology services, please visit us at www.nydermatologygroup.com, where you'll also find information on our new scientifically advanced and nutrient-rich Colbert MD skin care products line, Daily Nutrition for Skin.

———

For HSRD updates all year long, forever, visit: www.highschool reuniondiet.com.

Index

About the Authors

David A. Colbert, MD, founder and head physician of New York Dermatology Group in New York City, is board certified by the American Academy of Dermatology and board eligible in internal medicine. He has been established in private practice in Manhattan since 1993, after studying medicine at La Faculté Libre de Médecine in Lille, France, receiving his degree from New York Medical College, and completing his residency at Columbia-Presbyterian Hospital in New York. He is a member of the American Academy of Dermatology, the American College of Physicians and Surgeons, and the American College of Dermatological Surgeons.

Terry Reed is the author of several screenplays, including the independent feature and cult favorite *Cherry*, released in 2000. Her first novel, *The Full Cleveland*, was published by Simon & Schuster in 2005. She is currently writing a second novel and a book on nutrition for American teens. She has a master's degree in fiction and film from Columbia University.